ALTERED ON IMPACT
How a Traumatic Brain Injury
Taught Me to Lead a Purposeful Life

Lynn DelGaudio

ALTERED ON IMPACT: HOW A TRAUMATIC BRAIN INJURY TAUGHT ME TO LEAD A PURPOSEFUL LIFE

COPYRIGHT © 2019 BY LYNN DELGAUDIO

The content of this book is for general instruction only. Each person's physical, emotional, and spiritual condition is unique. The instruction in this book is not intended to replace or interrupt the reader's relationship with a physician or other professional. Please consult your doctor for matters pertaining to your specific health and diet.

To contact the author, lynndelgaudio@yahoo.com.

ISBN-13: 978-0-578-47271-3

Printed in the United States of America

LYNN DELGAUDIO, IHC

ALTERED

ON IMPACT

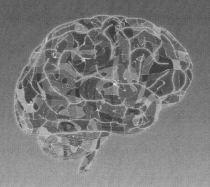

FROM TRAUMA TO TRANSFORMATION

*How a Traumatic Brain Injury
Taught Me to Lead a Purposeful Life*

PRAISE FOR ALTERED ON IMPACT

"All those folks who told you it's all in your head, well, guess what, it seems they may be right. Lynn DelGaudio has come out with this amazing book where she shares her personal story of how deciding and incorporating practices to change her mindset brought about a positive outcome to a life changing situation. These practices can be easily incorporated into your day-to-day routine, as seen in the stories she shares not only of herself but of her clients. This is a great resource for other health coaches who are working with clients to improve their health and wellbeing. Well worth your time to pick up this book and spend some days with it, as transformation doesn't happen overnight, to have your own mindset metamorphosis."

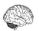 **Cheryl McPhee, Integrative Nutrition Certified Health Coach, CherylMcPheeWellness.com**

"What we perceive as reality often manifests as reality! In Altered on Impact, Lynn DelGaudio expertly reveals the impact of how tightly held belief systems can alter our perception of reality. DelGaudio's shared insights and roadmap for self-design will help all those who seek higher ground and more willful purpose in life. Those who choose to grow beyond their original DNA will recognize self as different from past programming or experience. DelGaudio suggests that to manifest a greater sense of wellbeing, a mindset metamorphosis is not only required but the inevitable outcome of an intentional process."

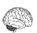 **Dr. Michael Fleischer, NewPathNutrition.com**

"Lynn's injury impacted her in a very unexpected yet glorious way. Rather than falling victim, she embraced her own creativity and power within, and has come out on the other side with such a highly positive light. Because Lynn experienced such a profound transformation within herself, she feels compelled to help others do the same. This is a great read about a remarkable journey."

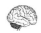 **J. Reilly Weed, RT(R)**

"By society's standards, DelGaudio has every right to be bitter and angry, to be a victim. She could have given up at any point in her journey, but she refused. She chose to create a better future for herself than what she was being told she would have. Her travels through life have not been easy, but through her own journey, she gives us the roadmap to become the best we can be without the limitations and restrictions that have been placed upon us. This book will inspire you and give you the tools necessary to change your life to be what you want it to be, but only if you put in the work. Don't wait for a catastrophe to decide it's time to be your best."

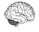 **Emily Fischer-Bunker, Integrative Nutrition Health Coach, JourneyToWellness.net**

DEDICATION

This book is dedicated to my many teachers along the way who have inspired me, educated me, guided and supported me, to those who have acted in integrity and inspired me through their actions, truth, will, and belief.

To Lisa, Lori, Mom, Dad, Barbara, Bobbi, Annie, Lynn, Terry, and anyone I've forgotten: All of you who just listened and let me vent, you have no idea how much that meant to me.

My beautiful, dear pooch and companion, Buddy: Thank you for finding me in this physical realm and being my best friend, unconditionally, every moment of every day of our time together! Your smile is indelibly marked in my mind!

And Reilly, thanks as always for your patience, understanding and humor! Little gestures of compassion and kindness can really make an impact in this world, and create their own current of continued acts of kindness.

"Success is no accident. It is hard work, perseverance, learning, studying, sacrifice, and most of all, love of what you are doing or learning to do."
-Pele

TABLE OF CONTENTS

PART I: THE JOURNEY OF MY INJURY

PART II: THE LEARNING OF A NEW SELF

PART I
The Journey of My Injury

CHAPTER ONE

IN AN INSTANT (everything changed)

"Choose to be optimistic, it feels better."
-Dalai Lama

July 3, 2014. On a beautiful, sunny, spectacular North Carolina day, I had just finished a great seven-mile run, and I was enjoying the high endorphin levels that came with it. This was a particularly good run for me: My form and strides were on point, my breathing was perfect and relaxed. My body felt great. Strong. Steady. Conditioned. Muscular. I was so grateful to be in such good running shape, and although a great workout, running was also always extremely meditative for me.

During my runs is when much of my creativity and insights were expressed, and all my stress released. This warm July day, I was feeling especially good. It was only noon and I had the entire afternoon ahead of me. I had nowhere to be, no work to do, and I was high on life. I was looking forward to the four-day July 4th holiday weekend and the great weather that the forecast was proposing. I was also looking forward to a trip to Connecticut the following week to see my family. It had been eight years since I had seen them, and I was so excited for the long overdue reunion.

Since I was in no hurry at all, I decided to lift some weights before taking my pooch for a walk in the nearby park. The community where I lived had a fitness center, so I headed over. I started with some behind-the-neck lat pull downs. I was strong. I was pulling seventy to eighty pounds on a given day at that time. I began. One...two..

In an instant, everything changed. I don't know if I finished the second pull, or if I had three or four pulls, or more. I don't remember much, except that I felt something snap and the bar came screeching down on my head with the force of seventy-five pounds. Upon impact, I literally felt my brain shake, like my head was a Christmas snow globe, swishing back and forth, and I saw a flash. I lifted my hand to feel my head and found a bump the size of a grapefruit, and it was growing fast. I felt to see if there was any blood...just a little, which might have been from the clip I had in my hair? The metal bar? I wasn't sure.

Being the day before a holiday, no one was present in the management office adjacent to the fitness center. I called a friend who worked as a radiology technologist in a local doctor's office. He advised me to call my primary care doctor, who was also a concussion specialist.

"Do you have the worst headache you've ever had?"

No.

"Are you nauseous?"

I don't think so.

"Well, our office is closing early and we are closed tomorrow for Fourth of July, so if either of those things happen, get yourself to a hospital immediately. We can get you in Saturday morning at 10:00 a.m."
At the suggestion of my friend, I just went back to my place and rested. *I feel weird, but I'll be okay,* I thought to myself. Thank God I was doing a rear pull down. If that had been a front pull down, I might have messed up my face, or even died.

I don't remember much of the next forty-eight hours, but I know I monitored myself. I kept the Saturday morning appointment. By that time, my symptoms were indicative of the blow to the head. When I entered the physician's office, I was quite off balance. My eyes were glazed over, my sight was blurred, and my speech was off. My doctor could tell I had a serious injury just by looking at me. At one point, my doctor left the room for a moment. I was experiencing such a bizarre feeling—I was fully aware that I wasn't fully aware. I felt so out of it, confused, disoriented. I turned and looked around the room. There was a countertop with some cabinets above. A computer sat on the countertop. There was a chair and exam table. "Where am I?" I looked back at the door, and, all of a sudden, I simply had no idea where I was. I tried to remember. I knew that I'd known where I was a minute ago, but then my sense of place and time abruptly left me. It was unsettling. When the doctor came back, I told her that I forgot where I was. I suppose she must have reminded me.

I don't remember much more about my visit, except that they made me do a bunch of "impact testing." These tests looked at things like spacial awareness and interpretation, recall, memory, reaction time, and a lot of other things that I can't even remember while writing this. One of the tests presented a series of different shapes, and then, after a brief pause, showed another series of shapes and asked me to answer whether or not each shape was the same from the first series? *What about this shape? This shape? Now this one?* What?! I had no idea. They were really hard! My inability to achieve anywhere close to a successful score, or to even finish the tests in the time allotted, was laughable. I was an otherwise very highly functioning professional—an individual who had always gotten As and Bs in school and graduated college with distinction—but I found these simple exercises nearly impossible. The test results showed cognition of only 0% to 5%. *Wow,* I thought. This was a new and very odd experience for me.

The doctor advised that I was to have no stimulation at all: no phone, no sound, no TV, no light, no nothing until further notice. But I was encouraged to walk ten minutes, twice a day—something about brain, motor, body, whatever connection. I was very unstable (vestibular and balance problems), so I could try to walk outside, or hang on to the railings of the treadmill if that felt safer.

In the days and weeks following the injury, my symptoms were increasing: double and blurred vision, blind spots, pain along the right side of my body, slurred and stuttered speech, headaches, and a *horrible* memory. If someone said something to me, it would be completely lost within a couple of seconds.

I also had a lot of compression in my cervical spine (C6-7, I think) that was causing a host of other problems, including tingling in the upper extremities, neck and shoulder spasms, and other random shooting pains.

Although I was told not to use my phone, I absolutely needed to call my boss to let him know what had happened. When he heard my sloppy speech and slurred words, he asked if I'd been medicating (I must have sounded drunk and it was 9:30 in the morning). I explained what had happened and that I'd be out of work for a few days. Immediately, he said, "Kiddo, this is gonna be a few weeks, not days." Little did either of us know, it would be even longer.

Friends and colleagues seemed to all have the same reaction: "Oh no! That's horrible! You must be so mad!" *Mad? Why would I be mad?* I didn't understand what anger had to do with anything. I wasn't even defining this "thing" as something horrible; only something that happened to me and that I was now experiencing, and that I would get through. I guess I just thought that I was experiencing some symptoms, but that I would be on the mend in no time. In retrospect, in those initial stages, the injury itself was keeping me from seeing the extent and seriousness of it all.

In the initial weeks following the injury, I spent most of my time laying either in my bed or on my couch. I'd just lay there all day. I got out of bed, freshened up, and transported myself from the bedroom to the living room couch. The living room was incredibly airy and bright, but I wasn't supposed to have too much light so I kept the shades drawn. Much of the time, my eyes were closed as well. In my catatonic, meditative state, I often heard, "bum 2 3, bum 2 3, bum bumbum… BUM… bum23, bum 2 3, bumbum, BUM… bum bum 2, bum 2 3, bum 2 3." I was more aware of my heart beating than ever before, and often heard an irregular beat. I was simply observing, not drawing any conclusion or attaching any meaning. At the time, I just thought, "Oh, that's a different beat."

I wasn't supposed to watch any TV. I turned it on once, I suppose because I didn't remember my doctor's instructions and just wanted to see the weather. As the screen came into focus, the meteorologist was describing an incoming weather system that was making its way from the west. The camera was panning from one side of the state to another, showing the track of the system. Woah… wuh… the dizziness made me feel like I was falling off of the couch. I covered my mouth, thinking the queasiness might result in an undesired tossing of breakfast. I quickly turned it off. Clearly, TV was not in the cards for a while; the movement of the screen was too problematic.

It wasn't just the TV, though. If I even turned my head left to right, just while standing, I'd become extremely dizzy and off balance, and often nauseous. I tried to stay close to walls (if I were to fall, I'd rather fall into a wall), and held on for dear life when stairs were involved. Stairs were frightening. The slope was incredibly challenging for my vestibular system, especially downslope.

On one of my two ten-minute required daily walks, my neighbor, Kenny, drove by and rolled down his window. "Are you okay?" My eyes were glazed. I was walking very slowly and off kilter. I told him what had happened. I had a really bad concussion. "Your eyes are all glazed over. You're not steady. Let me drive you home." (I was only fifty feet from home!) I got in the car and I that's all I can remember about that.

I was mush. Just. Mush.

Those were seemingly tough days, but I'd eventually come to know them as the easiest of all.

IMPACT IMPERATIVE #1
OBSERVATION/AWARENESS

You have to become an observer of your thoughts and feelings. Learning how to observe and increase your awareness is the first step in the learning process, and will help you develop the ability to pull more of your negative thoughts and beliefs out of your subconscious. This is done through still meditation as well as active practice. Meditation allows us to enter into the subconscious and become closer to our true self. The Tibetan word for meditation is Gom or Ghom, which means "to become familiar with your mind." The more we can become familiar with, gain knowledge about, embrace, and befriend all aspects of who we are, the more empowering and transformative the experience will be. Active practice using the tools outlined in this book is also important. Once we have gained our new awareness, we need to implement the proper tools to translate our new awareness, new knowledge, into a remarkable redesign.

CHAPTER TWO

BRAIN STRAIN (and learning to refrain)

*"Each day I come in with a positive attitude,
trying to get better."*
-Stefon Diggs

The funny thing about my brain injury was that as I began to heal, I became much more aware of the extent of the injury. As my brain began to repair and heal, it was actually registering more symptoms, and they were numerous: I still spoke with slurred and stuttered speech, suffered short and long term memory loss, headaches, internal head pressure, blind spots, dizziness, blurred and double vision, serious vestibular and balance issues, tinnitus, nausea, extreme confusion and disorientation, headaches, pain, trouble walking, trouble standing, impaired depth perception, and just about every symptom associated with such an injury. I now had a rash from head to toe that my dermatologist would later tell me was not uncommon after such traumas.

I also started to feel a weird electrical pain in my left calf from time to time, as well as a lot of low back pain. The neck and shoulder spasms and pain were worsening. I was now experiencing waves of pain from the back right toward the front right side of my head, and my eye pain was increasing.

After a couple of weeks of rest, my doctor instructed me to see a number of specialists on a regular basis: physical therapist, vestibular therapist, vision specialist, neurologist, speech therapist, and a traditional therapist as needed. I was to see each once or twice a week, in addition to my concussion check-ups. I also needed to see an ophthalmologist.

I was eventually cleared to drive ten miles per day, and I was allowed to incorporate light, people, and TV back into my world. I found, though, that I could barely watch any TV without getting nauseous and dizzy. Crowds and lights made me ill and anxious. Turning my head still made me nauseous and dizzy. From time to time, I forgot where I was, where I lived, and who people were. For example, I might run into someone who looked familiar, but I had no idea if they were a close friend, family member, acquaintance from the gym, or a barista at the local Starbucks.

From time to time, I said odd things. I would say, "Thank you," when someone sneezed, or I once told a friend that I needed to go buy cheese. I don't eat dairy. This bizarre behavior was unsettling. I felt highly unstable. I was nervous to be out in public because I was afraid that I might say or do something inappropriate. There really was no basis for this. I had said a couple weird things, but I hadn't done anything inappropriate in my healing process. Yet I routinely had thoughts like, *What if I decide to take my shirt off?* or, *What if I blurt out something nonsensical?* or, *What if I pee in public?* I tried to tell myself these thoughts weren't real, just thoughts.

The initial force to my head had rotated and tilted my neck, causing a host of issues in my cervical spine. The injury had impacted my occipital, parietal and temporal lobes. The occipital lobe is located at the back of the brain and controls sight. The parietal lobe rests in the middle region of the brain and relates to cognition, touch sensation (pain, pressure), and spacial awareness. The temporal lobe is located at the bottom section of the brain and manages memory, language, learning, emotion, hearing, and the interpretation and processing of auditory stimuli.

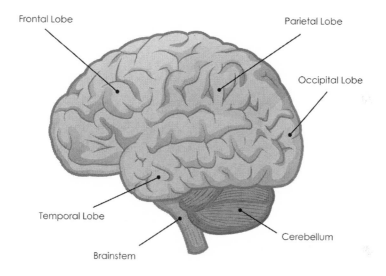

My vision was a disaster. I began seeing the eye specialist on August 11, 2014. This particular eye doctor, Dr. Peters, specialized in concussion and TBI related vision issues, and treated a number of professional athletes, especially professional hockey players. I felt very comfortable in his care. During those visits, I would wear goggles that distorted things a bit—no, a lot (at least in my brain and eyes)—and someone would toss a baseball to me. Right side first. Left side next. Center. I was retrieving far more lost balls than I was catching. It was difficult to catch any of those tosses the first visit. After a few months, I would attempt the same while balancing on a wobbly board.

Another exercise was kind of like Whack-a-Mole on the wall, but with lights that lit up instead of critters popping out of holes, and I'd have to tap them. It was dizzying, difficult, and it often took me hours to recover from the dizziness and nausea the exercises induced. But I viewed it as a fun game, as if I were a five-year-old. My "at home" exercises required I wear paper-framed glassed with plastic lenses, one lens red and one blue, while doing certain exercises. I don't have good recollection of these exercises. I just remember the glasses. By mid-September, 2014, Dr. Peters advised that he could no longer see me, at least for the time being. My vestibular issues were so significant that my vision would not correct properly until the vestibular imbalances were corrected.

The vestibular visits were starting to go a little better. My balance was improving, but I could not be on a treadmill at all without severe dizziness, which was so extreme, it was anxiety producing. After a while, they had to release me, saying there was nothing more they could do for me. I was at my new baseline. My new normal.

I returned to Dr. Peters, but it would be several months before my vision was restored to normal.

Meanwhile, co-pays for the specialist visits were about $1,600 a month. That was a big number, but I honestly didn't worry about it. I couldn't. It would've stressed me out if I let it, and that would've been counter to my healing. I was 100% committed to my healing, and I continued to see an assortment of doctors, all on a regular basis.

I needed help, though: rides to places, help with my dog, basic stuff. I had never been the type to seek assistance, and I took pride in being self-sufficient. That's all I knew. Even when I was married, my husband and I both traveled a lot for business and we were often home alone. I handled all the finances for us. I kept the house a home. I had always been, and still was a very independent, very private person. But I was quickly learning a great lesson from the injury. During my healing, people often said to me, as a way of consolation, I suppose, that God only gives you what you can handle. But I was learning, and would respond with my new-found revelation: "No. He gives you more, so that you ask for help." And I did. I had no choice.

Given my physical and neurological incompetence, I couldn't take good care of my dog. I certainly couldn't walk Buddy, as I was a considerable fall risk, and at the slightest tug of a leash, I'd likely do a head plant. Buddy is a sheltie-shepherd-retriever mix, and my best companion. I rescued him when he was about two years old. I was his fifth or sixth home. He had been abused and almost euthanized. When we first met, he was afraid of most sounds, would cower under any kind of shelter he could find—a chair, a table, a bed, or in a corner—and he never opened his mouth. He barked A LOT, and was afraid of men, especially tall men in hats. It just took some time, love, structure and a routine so that he knew he had a home. Buddy is always smiling. I feel like he was placed in my path to save me. Fortunately for me, one of the technicians at my dog's vet, which also had doggie day care, didn't live far from me. I asked her for help and she agreed without hesitation, with a wide open heart and a big smile. On some days, she would pick Buddy up in the morning and drop him back at night. Sometimes, she would take him to her place overnight so that I could rest, and let Buddy roam and play with her dogs. He loved those days! Other times, a friend or neighbor took care of him. The eagerness of friends and neighbors to help was beautiful, heartwarming.

A friend offered to take me to the grocery store a couple miles away. Other than doctor visits, it was my first excursion out of my house. We entered the store and it went well for the first few minutes. We made it through the produce section without incident. He needed cereal, so rather slowly (I wasn't walking too quickly yet), we made our way to the cereal aisle. He examined the selection of cereal choices and I continued down the aisle in amazement. I turned the corner between the cereal aisle and dairy section, and I became utterly paralyzed in awe as I gazed at all the colors on the boxes, containers, exploring the fonts on the food packages, the array of bright colors everywhere, and the magnitude of the available assortments and selections. I literally froze, stupefied. My friend saw me at the other end of the aisle, standing and staring, bewildered, and he came quickly. My eyes were glazed over with a dumb, half-smiling stare on my face. People were walking by me in all directions, and I just stood there, focused, but completely out of focus. "Okay, time to get going!" he said, and directed me out of the store and back to his car. We left without purchasing much. That was enough excitement for the day, possibly the week.

I tried to laugh at these situations, find the humor in them, because I knew I was safe, and I knew I'd eventually be okay. I guess I still had no idea how serious an injury I had sustained. And some of the stuff actually was comical. So, I prodded on and tried not to make any judgments about my condition. Through the whole process, I tried to be an observer and not attach any meaning to what I was experiencing. Still, my friends and colleagues continued to insist that I should be angry about this "thing" that happened to me, but I had no anger. I was deliberately choosing positivity.

About six weeks after the injury, in late August, 2014, I was cleared to work half days. Things seemed like they were improving, and on September 15th, I was cleared to work "as tolerated" with numerous mental breaks throughout the day. I was cleared to drive up to one hundred miles in a given day, but not on back to back days. By September 22nd, though, my symptoms were worsening substantially, and my driving was again restricted to no more than fifty miles per day, with no back to back days.

I was also instructed to take numerous mental breaks and limit activities that require a significant amount of attention or concentration. My job required both concentration and a lot of driving. However, driving now made me nauseous and dizzy, especially at higher speeds, so it took me much longer to get anywhere. Numerous times per trip, I had to pull over and wait until the dizziness or nausea passed enough for me to go on. Those stops typically took between five and twenty-five minutes. I had medication for the dizziness, but I tried not to use it, except for when my symptoms were severe. Though these meds didn't produce any side effects, I still hated to take them. I've always been that way about medication. I'd prefer not to use it if possible. My doctor wanted me to try medication for the headaches, but the side effects included skin rash, blurred vision, numbness and tingling. She suggested medication for the nausea, but that could produce dizziness and headaches. I thought, "Are you hearing yourself? How on earth does this make any sense or sound at all appealing? Those are the very symptoms I'm trying to ease!"

I was eager to get back to work, even if for partial work days, but the fifty-mile distance limitation meant I had to stay in hotels when my work required more than fifty miles in travel per day, which it often did. Add about $1,200 a month for hotel stays to the $1,600 a month in co-pays, and I was looking at around $2,800 a month in added expenses. Yikes. And that didn't even include *my portion* of $1,200 for the MRI, or Buddy's doggie day care, medications, other random tests and blood work. But again, I could not let this bother me. I had to maintain a positive outlook. Besides, it hurt my brain to do otherwise. It literally hurt to think of things that could potentially stress me out. I began to pay close attention to that. It seemed pretty simple: When I think stressful thoughts, I feel bad. When I think positive thoughts, I feel good. I preferred to feel good. Therefore, I began to think of good, positive thoughts as much as possible.

During the month of October, 2014, it seemed like I was taking one step forward and two steps back, then two steps forward and one step back, one step forward and three steps back. My impact test scores on October 24th were far lower than they were on August 13th. It made no sense. Or did it? The more I tried to return to work, the more stress I felt.

By November, 2014, I was still seeing a number of specialists: eye doctor, physical therapist, vestibular therapist, concussion specialist, neurologist, but I was now down to about five or six appointments per week.

My lack of any linear progression in my healing continued to frustrate me a bit, but I was determined not to be a victim. I began to pay more attention to my thoughts and reactions.

I was trying to not let the stress get to me. Consciously, I knew that giving my energy to worry would be taking energy away from healing. Subconsciously, if I was placing my attention and energy on the escalating debt, it would also take away from my healing. Either way, when stress reared her head, I would feel internal pressure in my skull, develop headaches, nausea, dizziness. Faced with any kind of stress at all, I would become symptomatic. The physical stress of staring at a computer or concentrating too long or hard, emotional stress of any kind, stress from mental or physical overexertion, stress from the mounting medical bills, which, thus far, already topped well over $20,000, not to mention the lost wages and other related expenses—it was all too much. The bottom line, though, did not change: I prefer to feel good. Not bad. It was that simple.

I had an epiphany. I began to understand three things very clearly: 1) *Whether or not I was conscious of it or not, I was thinking in fear.* 2) My thoughts can cause me stress and compromise my wellbeing, and 3) I have the ability to decide what thoughts I want to think. **I get to choose.**

In the days and weeks just after the injury, I was in silence in bed or on the couch, not thinking about much at all. Although it wasn't exactly meditation, I am convinced that there was an extraordinary meditative benefit. I now had an acute understanding that what and how I was thinking directly influenced how I was feeling and healing. I began to get very deliberate about paying attention to my thinking. I used active, deliberate, and directed thinking to assist in the healing process, because instead of letting a good feeling thought simply come into my mind, I was actually having fun choosing what I wanted to think about. Of course, I had my moments—many, many moments—where, in an instant, I would forget that I was even doing this practice. My memory issues were a bit of a hindrance, but I trekked on, without judgment, continuing my practice whenever it came into my consciousness, especially when I had some sort of somatic signaling, like tension in my neck or chest or a bad gut feeling. I have always been a firm believer that when there is an emotional or somatic response, it's worth looking into, as this is your body's way of conveying information to you.

I also decided that I would not allow negative people into my life, or at least I would chose to surround myself with positive people as much as I could. To the extent the negativity could not be avoided, well, then I would need to protect my brain and myself from it. The trick that worked best for me was to imagine a large bubble all around me, like the Michelin Man, and envision the negative energy pinging right off of the protective bubble. If I was able, I'd envision this bubble in advance of the interaction. I'd sometimes give it a color, like a light pink. And sometimes, depending on the person, I would envision a steel or hard plastic barrier that I could see through.

The decision to direct my thinking in a positive light was probably the first and most important step in my healing, as without that decision, there would've been no change. I was having fun devising the series of exercises to help me feel good, and was now trying to practice the following as consistently as possible: I was not judging and trying to see humor in awkward moments, choosing positivity at every turn, thinking positive and good feeling thoughts, being deliberate in choosing what I wanted to think about, paying attention to my body and somatic responses, and letting go of and protecting myself from the energy of negative people.

Little did I know at the time, these simple little exercises were not only helping me heal, but they would be the beginning of a road map that provided me a positive and sustainable plan for moving into an amazing future.

EXERCISES:

- Do you think about what you are thinking about? Try to start paying attention to your thoughts each day.

- Choose positive thoughts, and be deliberate about what you want to think about.

- Try to find humor in awkward moments and if you find you are judging yourself, give yourself a break.

- Pay attention to any somatic signals you might experience.

- Protect yourself from negative energy, try the Michelin Man exercise.

- Try these exercises each day for a week and keep a journal.

CHAPTER THREE

RAINDROPS ON ROSES (and other favorite things)

"Only in the darkness can you see the stars."
-Martin Luther King, Jr.

"I simply remember my favorite things, and then I don't feel *so bad!"* Who can forget that song, sung so beautifully by Julie Andrews in the brilliant musical *The Sound of Music*? The children were frightened by a severe thunderstorm, and by simply focusing their fearful thoughts on good thoughts and images, their individual and collective moods and energy instantly shifted. This line proposes one of the simplest examples of how to take control of our negative thoughts. Mental hygiene 101. And it works. I know, because it worked for me.

Equipped with my new revelation that a) my thoughts impact how I feel and b) I have a say in what I think about, I was ready to put this into practice. I developed a simple little exercise I called "My Favorite

Things." I had become really good at simply thinking good thoughts and keeping stress low, but now I was noticing that my stress was increasing, so I upped my game. Instead of just thinking good thoughts, I was now developing a good capacity for identifying negative thoughts and replacing them with my favorite positive thoughts instead. I would sit with the feeling just for a few seconds, just enough to notice, then let it go. I would then reach for something that produced a joyful feeling in me—running my toes through the sand while staring at the ocean, for example, was a favorite of mine, and still is. Then I'd sit with that for as long as possible. The energy shift was immediate and soothing. I started to get pretty good at this, and it was fun to do. One day while in practice, a memory from my childhood emerged:

One dreary, rainy day when I was a little girl, maybe eight years old or so, I was very upset, and staring out the window at the falling rain. It was a gray day and I was in a gray mood. Of course, I didn't know what triggered the sadness, but when my mom noticed my mood she said, "Okay, let's get your raincoat. Grab some of your crayons and colored chalk, too! I'll get the paper."

Suddenly, I was elated. I knew that we were going on some sort of adventure. My mom was taking control and would cheer me up. I sat in the backseat of the car with anticipation. The rain started to let up, widening our options. *Are we going to the park?* I thought. *A museum? Where could she be taking me?* We turned left off the main road in Farmington, Connecticut, the next town over from where I grew up. Other than the dreary, cloudy sky, it was a beautiful autumnal day, the New England foliage almost near peak, and I always enjoyed drives through this town and its country roads. I did not recognize this particular road, which was adorned with small farm houses and beautiful trees, boasting their bold fall-colored leaves.

As I gazed at the scenery, I noticed the car was slowing as we approached a relic of a graveyard—the historic kind where only thirty or so antique headstones remain. As the car continued to slow, I wondered why we might be stopping here for a bit. *Does Mom have a family member here that she wants to visit? Is it a short cut to another road?* She navigated the vehicle through a gate and pulled the car over. "Okay, bring your art supplies!" she said as she exited the front seat.

Confused, I slowly got out of the car, crayons and chalk in hand, paper securely rolled under my arm. My mother approached a gravestone and looked back at me, frozen in step. She waved me over and showed me the gravestone. "See," she said. "It says, 'I used to be, but am no more, at least in body mold. Yet shine do I and always will, at least that's what I'm told.'" Dismayed, yet curious, I slowly approached. At Mom's suggestion, I held the paper up to the stone and started to rub the chalk over the words so that the imprint of the words appeared as a poster on my paper. I looked down at my artwork. I thought, *What just happened?*

I had certainly forgotten my bad mood. That sad little girl that was staring out at the rain was long gone. My mother had made me forget completely about whatever it was that was creating a bad mood in me. Now, this was clearly a bizarre approach, but it worked. It was entirely effective. The experience piqued my curiosity about a lot of things (including my mother's psyche), and it made me forget the negative thoughts I was having. The point is that it's just that simple to replace negative thoughts with positive, or curious, even bizarre thoughts, very quickly. I continued to practice the "My Favorite Things" exercise as much as possible. I was certain this would help my brain heal.

It took about three months before I could get back to an exercise routine, but it wasn't *my* exercise routine. I couldn't run, and I had accepted that. I couldn't stay on an elliptical trainer for long, or walk on a treadmill, and I certainly could not ride a bike—the vestibular issues were still too much for me and I'd get dizzy and nauseous. But I could walk, so I did that as much as possible. I used that time to redirect my thoughts as much as possible. Walking became very meditative for me, just like running had once been. During my walks, I would think of things that made me feel good, and stay with the selected feeling, milk it, for as long as possible. I started to incorporate visualization as well. For example, I would visualize myself, fully healed and ridiculously happy. Over time, I began to notice how this practice of deliberately directing my thinking directly impacted how I felt. I don't know why or how I was coming up with these ideas. I was just glad I was, because they made me feel amazing.

During the healing process, I continued to notice how stress of any kind—negative thoughts, negative emotions, negative people, overexertion, anything stressful—directly and immediately impacted my brain and state of mind, and that continued to be of paramount importance to me. But despite this knowledge, I continued to feel increasingly irritable, fearful, insecure and panicky (also symptoms and consequences of the brain injury). I never felt angry, though others around me kept asking, "Aren't you mad? I would be so mad!" or, "Why aren't you mad?" or even saying, "You know, it's okay to be angry." I had to gently ask everyone around me to stop with this sentiment, as it was not at all helpful and counterproductive to my healing.

Of course, in retrospect, I see that my friends and colleagues instantly recognized the inevitable long and difficult trek ahead of me, but I had no concept of that "struggle" yet and, therefore, did not attach such a meaning to it, so on I went, facing each day as it came. Anger just never presented herself to me, but I was increasingly anxious and had experienced my first panic attack. I needed to do something. I just wasn't sure what.

New to the area in North Carolina, and having a career that required working remotely with significant travel, I had not yet established any supportive relationships, so it was entirely up to me and Buddy to get through this.

Although most people honored my request to keep their anger to themselves, I continued to hear from a few about how angry I "should be," as if somehow I should feel like a victim. But I didn't let that energy into my field. I couldn't. Something about the injury made me firmly declare I would NOT be victim to a simple circumstance of life. I clearly had a choice: to be angry, as some were suggesting, or to remain in a positive state of mind. The latter was without question more appealing, as not only was that the best approach to healing my brain and body, but it honestly just seemed more enjoyable. And most importantly, I knew I wasn't a victim and that somehow I would learn something from this experience.

But I couldn't seem to break through my new baseline. Although I wasn't angry, and as much as I tried to not to let things bother me, I was stressed. I was still highly symptomatic and my low back pain was worsening, as was the pain in my left calf. I continued to have moments of feeling scared, alone, sad, incredibly confused and highly anxious. Over time, the anxiety continued to increase significantly, producing profound and intense somatic responses and another panic attack. I knew I had to do something. I urgently needed to be more committed to my health, especially my brain and my mental health.

During the first several weeks following the injury, I was in a somewhat forced meditative state, so the more I healed, and the more I was allowed to work, drive, and get back to my physical routine and existence, the more anxiety I was experiencing. It made perfect sense to me that I should attempt to maintain a meditation practice through the healing.

Meditation is the practice of quieting and calming the mind, and letting go of active thinking. There is fear-based overstimulation everywhere with breaking news, high alerts, natural disasters, and we face a variety of stressors in our lives—environmental, physical, and emotional. Over arousal in the brain has been associated with a host of disorders from anxiety to poor sleep and depression. Poor diet, lack of exercise, stress, pollution, trauma—all of these things and more can send our brainwaves out of balance. When we change our thoughts, we change our perceptions and our brainwaves. I cannot stress enough the importance and impact meditation has had for me during this process. Like many of the tools in this book, it can be done anytime and anywhere, has no cost but provides substantial benefits, and does not require a huge time commitment.

I first started meditating with purpose in my early thirties, and I was fairly disciplined about it. I moved around a lot, and had already lived in three countries, eight states, and countless cities and towns. But no matter where I was living, I always made sure that I had one or two areas or rooms that were reserved, at least in part, to my yoga and meditation practice. I made sure that these were relaxing environments and they usually always had a fountain running and some natural bamboo plants. These areas contained a certain energy, and simply stepping into them, into their energy, brought me into a calm state. Like many, I would meditate regularly with discipline for several months or a couple of years, and then fall out of practice until some stress-inducing event occurred in my life that compelled me to start practicing again. But I could always enter my reserved meditation spaces and immediately feel the energy of peace and calm. It's similar to muscle memory when you haven't ridden a bike for years, and then one day you get on a bike and your muscles say, "Oh yeah! I remember this!" So it is for me when I return to my meditation practice and my mind says, "Oh, hello! So happy to see you again!"

I have always been at my best, most creative, and most calm when successfully practicing meditation on a daily basis. I've done a few different types of meditation in the past, but during this healing, I opted for simple Zen meditations, where I would sit or lay comfortably, close my eyes, and focus on my breath, breathing through my nose. I would notice any thoughts as they drifted through my mind and let them go, redirecting my attention to my breath. I meditated at least once a day for at least ten minutes to start, and then at least twenty minutes, then thirty. I attempted to maintain my daily practice as best I could, and vowed that when I did return to work, I would not let that interfere with the practice. My meditative state quite literally became one of my favorite things.

EXERCISE:

- Try noticing when a negative thought comes to mind, or when you have a negative reaction to something. Then, identify the thought(s) that preceded the reaction. Begin to think about your favorite things (running your toes through the sand, a puppy in your arms, your love, whatever it is), and notice the difference. How do you feel? Journal.

CHAPTER FOUR

YEAH, I'M FINE (I think?)

"Right now, I'm having amnesia and deja vu at the same time. I think I've forgotten this before."
-Steven Wright

December of 2014, I was finally cleared to work full time again. When I first returned to work, I was still bouncing into walls, walking unsteadily, and I'm sure I seemed quiet or different in some way; at least I felt quiet and different. I worked for a bank in the capacity of a Special Assets Officer. This position deals with the "bad debt" of the bank. When a borrower defaults on their debt, say a shopping center or subdivision, the Special Assets Officer needs to make a decision as to how to proceed in a way that will best protect the bank's interest. That strategy, in general, usually takes one of three forms: litigation, foreclosure, re-structure/workout, or perhaps a combination thereof. It can be an incredibly stressful job at times for several reasons, not the least of which is you are constantly giving bad news to people. These professionals are the busiest after an economic downturn, and the job requires a mixture of analytical, investigative and creative problem solving skills. You must possess a sound understanding of real estate and legal concepts and procedures. It also takes a strong personality to be in this role. You must be tough, firm, possess a strong backbone and not allow the emotions or statements of the borrower impact your duties, your effectiveness.

I've always struggled with the human aspect. Some borrowers have just lost everything—their entire empire, entire savings and retirement. Sometimes, they are simply wiped out, deflated, even sick because of it. They are hurting, yet we have a job to do. I have always tried to use compassion in my dealings, but I had a job to do. For the most part, people are understanding, but, from time to time, a borrower who has lost a lot can react unpredictably, and that's when this role can become a little unpredictable, dangerous even, though thankfully not often. (In the past ten years, I've had my life threatened a number of times, once with a Glock 43X to my temple.)

Back in 2013, I had to negotiate a settlement with a borrower who had lost his real estate empire and almost all of his retirement. He was in his early seventies. We negotiated a small settlement (the bank had written down the debt to $0.00, so anything would have been a recovery). He was out of state, and the settlement was negotiated entirely over the phone and email. Several months later, he was at a local branch where I was holding a meeting. A loan officer called me over to meet him in person. I was so nervous. The borrower first shook my hand and then gave me a hug and thanked me. "You're thanking me? Why?" I asked. He said kindly, "I didn't always like what you said, Lynn, but I always admired you for how you said it. You know, I lost everything. All I have now is my wife, a beat up RV, and a nice bottle of red wine at night. You know, it took me all these years to realize that that's all I really need. Life is so simple now. Thank you." I stared for a moment. I tried to hold the tears back as he offered me another hug, which I accepted. I never saw or heard from him again, but to this day, I wonder how he and his wife are doing.

The position requires constant documentation review and financial analysis. A math geek myself with an accounting degree, I was always highly analytical. I enjoyed crunching numbers, it came fairly easily to me. DiffyQs (differential equations) were fun for me, and I can still recite the quadratic equation. Growing up, I was very good with grammar and verbal communication, but reading was very difficult for me. I didn't know about dyslexia much back then, and it typically took me two to four hours to complete reading assignments that my friends easily finished in one hour. My mother nonchalantly mentioned to me when I was twenty-eight that she was so glad I got over my dyslexia. She and my father decided not to tell me when I was young because they didn't want me to feel "less than." They also saw what a hard worker I was, and figured that trait would serve me well in the future. So I just studied very hard at everything, but math and I were great friends with little struggle.

So there I was, back at work, falling into walls (pretending I was just leaning and reviewing a document), getting tripped up on my words, not remembering what people had just said (but nodding as if I did), and, apparently, forgetting who people were. In my journal, I wrote the following:

12/9/14 -

Upon returning to work today, there was a function in the training room, and people were congregating in the kitchen on a break. I approached a woman and introduced myself. "Hi, I'm Lynn. I know we've seen each other, but I don't think we've actually met," to which she responded, "Lynn! Hello! Nancy... the CFO, remember?!" Embarrassing!!! I knew her and, in fact, had attended meetings with her every month!!

From time to time, I was asked, "Are you sure you should be here?" or, "Are you sure you should be driving?" or, "Are you sure you're okay?" Yeah, I was fine. Just a little wobbly and foggy still, but certainly my doctor would not allow me to return to work if she did not feel confident in that decision. So, on I trudged. My boss, Richard, had taken care of things in my absence, bless him. But now, it was time for me to retake the reins. It didn't take me long, maybe a day, to realize this was going to be difficult.

On the first day of my return, Richard was trying to reconcile an enormous spreadsheet full of complicated macros and calculations. Reconciling and integrity checking wasn't necessarily a difficult process, but it was extremely tedious and time consuming. I jumped right in to assist. The eye strain first hit after about fifteen minutes, but I kept going. After about forty-five minutes, though, I felt my head fill with pressure and I got a nasty headache. He could see it in my eyes, turned and said, "Okay, time for a break, kiddo,"

The days continued on like that—work for a bit, recover for a while. I could only look at detailed spreadsheets or a computer screen for short periods. When I started to delve back into the debt re-structures, I realized that I had no recollection of some fundamental concepts. *What exactly constituted a TDR (troubled debt restructure)? What earned a credit "non-accrual" status?* These are really basic concepts that I simply could not recall. I started to realize that I had actually forgotten some of the basic fundamental concepts and processes of my job. Outwardly, I looked very normal, and people expected me to be just as normal on the inside. But I wasn't. Not even close. And I couldn't let anyone know. The problem was that I needed to do enough to make everyone believe that I knew what I was doing, yet not do too much for fear of "re-concussing" myself. I assumed folks would cut me a little slack for having suffered such an injury, but not for long. For months, I would have to dance a very delicate dance, attempting to slowly re-learn the fundamentals of my job, while also paying very close attention to my brain. If I concentrated too hard or for too long, I would get nauseous, dizzy, develop a headache, vision issues, and head pressure. It was extremely difficult navigating through those waters.

Not long after my return, something curious started to happen. I began to be uninvited to executive and board meetings, uninvited to a variety of meetings in which I had routinely participated. At one point, I expressed my concern to Richard, mentioning that if they are thinking of firing me, they'd better think again. That would be a wrongful discharge and I'd sue.

Richard was being promoted to Chief Credit Officer in the first quarter of 2015 and he was more than deserving. In late January, 2015, he was called to the CEO's office, and he assumed it was to discuss the details of the promotion. Instead, they gave him six months to leave. It made no sense. He was devastated. Worse still, I was to eventually take his place. This was such a complete and severe injustice. I was angry, as well as terrified.

Richard was such a mentor to me, and just a fun person to be around. He is one of the brightest people I've ever known, and very down to earth. He built an incredibly cohesive team at the bank; we were a well-oiled machine. I would now inherit the team. In my heart of hearts, I knew I didn't want the responsibility. It had been many years since I managed a group of people, and frankly, I wasn't interested. But it was a paycheck, and a good one. God knows I needed it with the medical bills piling up. I was not at my boss's caliber—he was lightyears beyond me, technically and intellectually—and I knew how much the group liked and looked up to him. They barely knew me. In fact, the bank was actually a client of mine when I was an independent consultant after the 2008 downturn. Our team assisted regional community banks find merger partners and/or acted as a special assets department until the banks could develop one on their own. Eventually, this bank hired me as a full-time employee, but I had only been a FTE for six months before the injury, and I was mostly on the road. So the team didn't really know much about me other than who I was with my injury.

I was stressed. How on earth would I be able to fill this role when I can't even remember how to do my job? On top of that, I felt guilty about Richard's departure. Did I cause that? In the Special Assets world, our role is to clean up the bad debt, and as the bad debt shrinks, so, too, does head count. A CEO simply can't keep the same salaries in the budget. I was keenly aware of this, and also acutely aware of my mounting medical bills. With that in mind, in mid-January, I requested a one-on-one meeting with the CEO and asked him straight up what the landscape looked like for me. He was quite candid and told me that, at some point, one of us, either Richard or I, would have to go. A couple of weeks later, Richard was put on notice.

CHAPTER FIVE

BETTERING BRAIN (and worsening pain)

"Patience is not the ability to wait, but the ability to keep a good attitude while waiting."
-Joyce Meyer

Upon arriving at this very point in the process of writing this book, I felt somewhat drained, deflated, paralyzed, a bit unimaginative, uninspired, fatigued, with an enormous writer's block. I had been moving along with some ease to this point, so what changed? Since I'm all about examining my thinking, I checked in with that. *What was I just thinking or expressing before this point?* And it was an interesting answer. The previous chapter had been all about my work experience.

Work had become a massive drain, and I was beginning to feel incredibly unsatisfied within my career. Was it the career, though, or something else? If I dissect the events of the last several months, it is clear that thinking about work, my job, brought with it a host of other negative thoughts: the dizziness and nausea while driving, the head pressure, headaches, nausea and eye pain when concentrating or staring at a computer screen, the failure to recall fundamental elements of my job (and interesting that I chose the word "failure"), the future role that I did not want but felt I had to accept, the stuttering while speaking, and on and on and on.

Maybe it wasn't the work at all, just my thoughts about it. Regardless of my attempts to remain in an emotional and mental state of wellbeing, despite all my efforts to get my mind and body in balance, and even in spite of how far I had come since July of 2014, it seemed that my negative internal narrative was now triumphing, or maybe I was just becoming more aware of or resisting the narrative. My pain, on the other hand, was most definitely taking the lead.

By March of 2015, eight months after the initial injury, I was still seeing the speech, eye and concussion doctors, but I had been released by all the other specialists who had determined that they'd gotten as far as they could with me. I still had some serious vestibular issues, but I would simply have to adjust to a new normal. *Will I ever be able to ride a bike again? Will the remaining imbalances work themselves out?* I felt 100% certain that I would never again be able to run on a treadmill. The dizziness was so significant and anxiety producing. I was okay with that. In the grand scheme of things, running on a treadmill is trivial, insignificant.

Will my back ever feel better? And what of the shocking, electrical and breathtaking left calf pain? It was steadily intensifying as the days and weeks went on. I had originally mentioned this to my doctor two weeks after the injury. "That's weird. You're just getting older, I guess," would be her mantra. It was so incredibly frustrating, but I knew something wasn't right, so I continued to try to get answers. I was full of optimism each time I made an appointment with a new doctor, proclaiming, "They'll get to the bottom of it! I just know it!" But still, no one had. I felt deflated every time I left a new physician's office.

The way I was experiencing life and the vision I had of my future were so drastically changed in an instant. I was vibrant, healthy, highly functioning. I was a successful professional, athletic, happy, vivacious, and I was looking forward to traveling and exploring the mountains, small towns, and coastal areas of the state. That was my original goal for the coming year. Now, I was a broken fifty-year-old woman, feeling elderly and concerned about the prospects of a far-less-than-full recovery, both mentally and physically. I had seen an army of doctors with an assortment of specialties, but it seemed all the king's horses and men just could not put me back together again. According to a couple healthcare providers, there was a strong possibility that I would have neurological, orthopedic and musculoskeletal issues for several years, if not for the remainder of my life. I continued to see my chiropractor, and found a new physical thera- pist and tried to work in regular massages—I thought it might help relieve the pain I was still in. Although I was feeling blue over my physical state, I still had some energy and the will to continue to find answers.

Work seemed to be getting a little easier, and I had no restrictions, so I could now drive as needed without limitations. I continued, though, to feel like I was operating at only fifty or sixty percent of my abilities, both physically and intellectually. I got confused a lot still, and I contin- ued to stutter when speaking at times. I continued to have substantial low back pain, which interfered with the regular course of business. At meetings, I would squirm in my chair every minute or so as it was painful to sit for any period of time. Driving wasn't as bad as sitting in an uncom- fortable office chair, but when driving any distance to speak of, I often had to pull over and stretch for several minutes.

And the calf pain frightened me. If I was standing when it hit, I would fall to my knees. If it hit while driving, there was no telling if I'd be able to control the wheel. If it hit while walking down the stairs (difficult enough without this complication, due to the continued vestibular issues), then I could topple down if I wasn't holding on to a railing. Walking up and down stairs was dizzying and felt precarious, dangerous. I often had to visit attorney's offices to discuss legal matters relative to my Special Assets job. One particular attorney had concrete stairs leading to the front door, and no railing. I was terrified each time I had to ascend and descend.

Compared to my condition seven months prior, my TBI symptoms were now showing some substantial improvement. But despite the improved condition and my practice of deliberate positive thinking, I still felt uninspired, uneasy, angst-ridden. I was still clearly consumed by uncertainty, worry, concern, and now, a new emotion: disappointment. I was disappointed this had happened, disappointed in my primary care doctor, disappointed that no one could "fix" me, but mostly, I was disappointed that I could not find the answers within myself.

In February of 2015, my sister, Lisa, came into town to visit. It was a Saturday evening, and we were just hanging out, figuring out what to do for dinner. We decided to go out to a local restaurant, Firebirds. We sat in the bar area at a high top and ordered some appetizers. I was a little dizzy, but not bad.

A woman approached, "Hey, Lynn! Where've you been?" I looked at the woman, briefly shifted my eyes over to Lisa, puzzled, and then back at the woman. "I'm sorry. I had a head injury and I don't have the best memory." She offered an understanding look and said, "It's Karen. From the gym." OH, my goodness! Of course I knew Karen! How embarrassing. She was kind and understanding. Our greeting was brief before she returned to her table of friends. The bar began to get crowded and the music was getting louder. I became extremely nauseous and dizzy and we had to leave.

Over several months, it became clear that I lacked relationships in my life. So, still suffering from continued pain and symptoms, I desperately attempted to regain any semblance of a personal life, to make connections, even go on a date. Steve was the general manager of the gym where I worked out, and he was also a friend. He knew all about my injury and was very supportive. He also had a crush on me and had asked me out on several occasions. It took me a while, but I ultimately agreed and we finally went out in March. But again, the headache, dizziness and nausea quickly ensued, and we had to cut it short after only thirty minutes. This was now getting a little irritating. *How long was it going to take? It's been eight months!* My social life would clearly be placed on hold for the time being. I needed to be patient and let this unfold however it was going to unfold. I continued to simply focus on my healing and my job. During the month of March, the calf pain seemed to be improving slightly and I began to wonder if it was subsiding for good. *Am I done with it? Is it done with me?* I was hopeful.

By April, the electrical pain came back with a vengeance, worse than ever. It certainly was not done with me. I was visiting an assisted living facility that the bank was taking back as part of a foreclosure. I was planning on flying to Connecticut the next day to see my family (the trip that, a year ago, had been suddenly postponed). I suddenly felt a sharp pain in my chest. I didn't think much of it, but it began getting worse, and I was having difficulty breathing. I was about an hour away from my doctor, so I thought about going to urgent care, but I didn't. I just wanted to see my doctor. While they were evaluating my chest and lungs, the electrical pain in my left calf was making itself known in a big way. It was so sharp, it took my breath away, and I screamed. She looked at me, concerned, and asked how long it had been going on. "Remember? Since right after the injury," I said. She said she needed to order more tests. I asked if those could be done the same day, as I was getting on a plane the next day to head north. "Oh no, you're not getting on any plane. You need to go to the hospital immediately," the doctor said she was concerned that I might be experiencing a pulmonary embolism, and off I went to the hospital to be tested. I did not have a PE, just pleurisy. But once again, my trip north was canceled in an instant.

By the summer of 2015, the demands of my work were increasing. I was on the road a ton. I would be officially taking over Richard's job in September. I still didn't know how I was going to handle it. I wasn't 100% in my ability yet (not even close!), my vision had still not corrected, and my pain continued to worsen. I had been journaling since the injury last July, and I wrote the following in my journal in June, 2015:

> *I continue to feel pain in my low back, a pinching in my thoracic area and stiffness/spasms in my neck. I also have tightness in the hips, and recently, the pain in the calf has begun to impact the left thigh. This pain is horrifying and it frightens me. I have recurring tingling and some numbness in the feet, predominantly on the right side. My hands have also experienced tingling, again, predominantly on the right, and about a week ago, my right hand froze and I was unable to move it. This happens occasionally and lasts for a few hours, on and off. There is no coincidence that all of this began with the head injury and it seems bizarre that no one can get to the bottom of it!*

By August of 2015, my vision finally seemed to be back to normal and my eye specialist gave me a big thumbs up. Otherwise, my recovery was about as good as it was going to get. I continued to work on my thinking, but the physical pain was too strong for my mind.

My leg pain was getting worse each day that passed. I was increasingly alarmed and concerned. At this point, patience was becoming utterly critical.

EXERCISES:

- How do you feel about your work? Relationships? What story are you telling yourself about these areas?
- Have you ever experienced pain that interfered with your positive thinking? What did you do?

Journal your experiences.

CHAPTER SIX

DEMONIZED & DEFEATED (Pain: 10, Lynn: 0)

"Your pain is an opportunity to learn about yourself."
-Gary Zukav

In late September of 2015, work really heated up and I was in charge of a large note sale for the bank. It was a lot of work, but I was good at this. I enjoyed it. This was all number crunching and my team was rock solid at getting these transactions accomplished. It was also an opportunity for me to shine and show the C-level executives that I could handle the new role. The timeline was very tight, and the deadline was Thursday, November 19th, the week before Thanksgiving. My leg pain continued and I just dealt with it. I kept telling myself that I just needed to get over the finish line of this transaction, and then I would find **someone** who could figure this out. By this time, I was in pain every minute of every day. The pain took my breath away. I had been to several different doctors and no one had a clue what was causing all the pain.

My office was almost ninety minutes away. On November 17th, 2015, two days prior to the closing of the note sale, I checked into a hotel so that I could just work late and get to the office the next couple of days without the long drive. By now, my leg pain occurred frequently throughout the day, in fact, many times an hour, and I was afraid to drive, so I was staying in hotels often.

I arrived at the office at 7:30 a.m. and the pain was excruciating. Without warning or conscious thought, I would scream when it hit. I advised my team ahead of time that they would likely hear me screaming. "I'm okay, though. It's just that the pain comes so quickly and is so intense, it just sends me screaming and takes my breath away. I don't have any time to adjust." They must have thought I was absolutely nuts to put work first rather than my health but we were very close to the closing, no one else could take my place on this assignment, and I'd already been to eight doctors and no one could figure it out. So, I continued on as best I could. An entry in my journal describes my pain at the time:

> 11/17/15:
> I feel like an 80-year-old and am tired of being told that it's just because I'm getting older. It is clear that something is wrong. Pain levels vary depending upon the area of pain. On a 1-10 scale, the back pain morphs between a 4-5 at its best to 9-10 at its worst. The shooting pain to the left calf, on the same scale, is about a 50. It's agonizing, unrelenting, exhausting and terrifying. I live in fear every day now and am exhausted living life this way.

By 11:00 a.m., I could no longer stand the pain and decided to head back to the hotel to get some rest. I was in extraordinary agony, but it was a quick drive to the hotel. The hotel was just a block or so, the second right after getting off the highway. Unfortunately, I was so disoriented by the pain that I took the first right instead. The first right was the exit ramp for Interstate 95 and I was heading onto the highway in the wrong direction. I saw a few cars pass me, pointing out their windows at me, as if to say, "What are you doing?!" Emotionless, I turned around safely, and headed to the hotel.

Once I got to my room, the pain was so severe and relentless, I thought it best to check out and go home—whatever little items still needed to be handled, I knew my staff could take care of it. I had planned on staying in town one more day, but this was too serious and I needed to get to a doctor or hospital or something. I decided to take a quick shower first, and while in the shower, something horrifying happened. If I moved my head even a couple of degrees, electrical pain shot down through my body into my left calf, rendering me a wild animal, screaming in pain. I couldn't move at all without being electrocuted repeatedly. The pain was unimaginable. It was the most terrifying, hopeless, helpless and desperate feeling. To this day, I don't know or remember how I got my things into the lobby—I honestly don't—but when I did, Lynn, the general manager saw me and ran to my side. "Where are you going?" she asked. "Home," I replied. "No. You cannot. What is wrong?" she urged.

Clearly the pain showed on my face and in my posture and body language. I explained my pain. I needed to go home. The staff at the hotel, bless them, jumped into action. Two of the staff drove me ninety minutes back home to ensure I got there safely. Blaire, a front desk manager and also a nursing student about to graduate and take boards, drove my car (I reclined in the passenger seat). Larry, a maintenance worker, followed in his car. We stopped by my office to pick up some paperwork. My team was perplexed. *Who were these people and why were they escorting me here and then home? What was going on?* My pain level was so high, I didn't have time to explain.

I phoned my doctor on the way home, screaming from time to time, and she ordered a prednisone pack to my local pharmacy. I was trying to breathe deeply and use visualization to help the pain. Blaire was telling me stories of her childhood—a nurse in practice. She was amazing! An angel sent to me right in the very moment I needed her. Larry was there all along in the rear view. They were both good drivers. We went back roads, even though it would take a little longer, it was a pretty and peaceful drive, and in my state, the less stress, the better.

We arrived at the pharmacy drive-through at 1:30 p.m. and picked up the prednisone prescription. The pharmacist advised that I should take the first six tablets as soon as possible. I grabbed my water bottle and downed the first six. Blaire and Larry dropped me off and saw that I got in my place safely. I will never forget their unbelievable gesture. I made sure to write a letter to InterContinental Hotels Group praising them for going WAY out of their way to help, and I made sure I gave them, and Lynn, the GM, a nice Christmas gift. Wherever you three are, I'll never forget that day.

My niece, Marisa, was living with me at the time. Marisa is my sister Lisa's daughter. She and her brother, Louie, are my only niece and nephew, and they are remarkable young individuals. Marisa had originally come to North Carolina in 2010 to attend UNC at Chapel Hill. Like her aunt, Marisa has always had an affinity for all things Spanish. She and I both spent time in Sevilla, Spain during our college years. Marisa graduated with distinction from UNC with a double major in Spanish and Exercise Science. She had just returned from a second trip to Spain, this time to live in Rhonda, a beautiful mountaintop town in the Andalucia region.

Marisa came home shortly after 3:00 p.m. and heard me screaming in the bathroom. The prednisone was not yet helping with the pain. My screams were now only minutes or less, sometimes seconds, apart. I was reduced to a writhing, tormented animal, shrieking in pain. My poor niece didn't know what to do. At 3:30 p.m., the medicine was not yet working. Still screaming. Continual torture by electrocution. 4:00 p.m., no relief. 4:30 p.m., an absolute feeling of terror washed over me, as if I was possessed and would require an exorcism. The pain was hitting every sixty seconds or less. My neck and throat hurt from screaming at such a loud decibel. I was entirely out of breath; each strike took my breath away so quickly and harshly that I felt I'd just run a hundred-yard sprint or four-minute mile. I was disoriented. Defeated. I'd had it. I didn't know what to do. The only alcohol I ever consumed was wine, and it would never have entered my mind to drink during the day, but I didn't know what to do. The one thing I knew was that this pain was no longer bearable. I couldn't go on like this. I opened a bottle of wine and had a glass. And another. And a third. And now, I was a terrorized, possessed and tormented animal, writhing in pain, with a wine buzz.

Around 5:00 p.m., we headed to the hospital. The doctors gave me something and tried to ask me questions, but it was nearly impossible for me to answer. I would scream so loudly that all of North Carolina probably heard. I would then need to take some time to recover and catch my breath in between electrocutions, as the shrieking took so much out of me. I was so exhausted and disoriented that just as soon as the doctor asked a question, I forgot what he had just said. I was 100% in survival mode now and could not respond to anything but my own attempt to endure and exist another minute in my body. My niece attempted to answer the questions for me, but the doctor insisted he hear from me. I did my best. The doctor was incredibly rude as I recall, and, in fact, accused me of being in the hospital to score drugs. I couldn't let it affect me, but I suppose on some level it did. On the way out of the emergency room, a nurse consoled me, indicating she knew that shriek very well, nerve pain. It was horrible. I had a prescription for a low dose of Gabapentin for the nerve pain, which seemed to work well, for the time being anyway.

During the very early morning on November 18th, I woke with double vision and blind spots on my right eye, and later that day, my vision was still off and I developed a headache. I first thought that this might be post-concussion syndrome again, but it was likely a side effect of the Gabapentin. I wrote the following in my journal:

> "I don't feel safe, and I'm extremely concerned about my wellbeing. I let work know that I will be out the balance of the week and spoke with HR and my boss about the latest developments."

Later that day, I met with a doctor at a pain management center. I was in such pain walking into her office. She was extremely professional, clear minded, thoughtful in her questions and responses, and I felt like I was in good hands. At the end of the exam, she asked if there was any ongoing litigation and I said there was, to which she simply replied, "Okay." I thanked her for not turning me away. "Why would I do that?" she asked. I explained that I had already been turned away by four doctors due to the litigation. "I wouldn't do that," she offered. "Do you think you can help me?" I asked, nervous for her answer. "Yes. I can," she replied. I cried uncontrollably. We set an appointment for me to come back for an epidural. That would be the first in a series of several epidurals.

I had left my chiropractor a message about my hospital adventure and he called that night to see how I was doing. I told him that I was fearful there was something serious going on in my spine, I was fearful to be alone, fearful the nerve pain would return, even fearful I would be paralyzed. His response was, "Well, clearly, there is some shifting going on in the lumbar spine in the vertebrae or disc and the pain you are experiencing is the classic tale of a ruptured disc or shifting, and while paralysis is possible, it is highly unlikely." I suppose I would have preferred to hear, "That's not going to happen, so just put it out of your mind." I tried my best to keep this out of my mind, but it was difficult. I was now existing in a constant state of fear.

11/18/15: It's been a long couple of days. Having good relief from the Gabapentin and was able to sleep through the night. I have been thinking a lot about work. I am unable to drive any distance for the foreseeable future, and that type of driving, though a requirement for work, is dangerous given my condition. My fear, which becomes more and more a reality as time goes on, is that I will need to find another career path (at 51! right!), as I am now unable to complete the duties required (driving to collateral, clients, etc.). My lifestyle will necessarily change, as I will not be able to earn the level of income I now do. This is awful to contemplate. I try not to put too much energy into it, as I need to focus on healing and wellbeing. The last two days have worn me out. I am amazed that I even made it through the nerve pain I experienced. I am physically and emotionally drained.

11/21/15 - Worried I will never be able to drive to the office, given the distance, or any other distances for work (or pleasure, for that matter). Afraid to change leg position much for fear excruciating nerve pain will return. Afraid there is nerve damage unseen/unknown as of yet. Nervous about a lot all of a sudden. I've never felt like this before, so full of fear. Had more x-rays today. If I have any more radiation, I will start to glow in the dark!

11/22/15 - Felt better this morning. Slept very well. Still have some pain in left calf, but nothing like the past week!!! Then in the afternoon, went grocery shopping with my niece. In the middle of the store, screamed as pain in left calf came on suddenly. Afraid to drive, gave keys to Marisa. Afraid to walk or do anything for fear horrific pain will return and not stop. Beautiful sunny day - normally would be taking a walk but am afraid to. Is this how my life is going to be? What will happen to my livelihood if I cannot drive? That is a big part of my job! They will likely let me go. I thought the epidural would take care of this pain.

Over time, the Gabapentin was not working well. I continued to experience sharp electrical pain in my left calf, and now the left knee, as well as dull pain, throbbing and numbness along my right leg and foot. I was not sleeping well at all. I was extraordinarily tired, and I'd stopped taking walks altogether, but I walked in my mind—in imaginary places I could go to and visualize a healthy me walking, smiling. I was able to go to those places for a few minutes or more, before... BOOM! being snapped back to reality and the horrible pain that had become my shadow, had become ME!

A student my entire life of the power of the mind, clearly I could go beyond my pain, I could train my brain around it. I've walked on coals for goodness sake! Coals were no match for this. I've had a gun to my temple twice and once the trigger pulled. (When I was eight years old, a man held a gun to my head and, before he pulled the trigger, said, "Don't worry, it's not loaded.") This was more terrifying than all of those experiences. I was feeling lost. I could not work. I could not play. I tried to be outwardly appropriate, outwardly pleasant and cheerful, but internally, I was suffering. I was suffering horribly. I could not stay out of pain long enough to feel good, feel happy, even for a few minutes. It was perplexing because after the initial injury, even though symptomatic, I was still pretty happy. Too happy to some, in fact. Yet in the last number of months, the pain had stolen my power. The pain had stolen Lynn.

CHAPTER SEVEN

IT'S THE MOST ~~WONDER~~**PAIN**FUL TIME OF YEAR

"Everything you want is on the other side of fear."
-Jack Canfield

Iusually put the tree up well before Thanksgiving so that I can enjoy the magic of a well-lit and decorated tree for several weeks. At Thanksgiving, my niece and I adopted a practice of cooking a few salmon, a huge turkey, a bunch of side dishes, and feeding the homeless we had come to know. We would also bring water and pie and some clothing or whatever we noticed one might be in need of. Wayne made a special impact on us. He was a veteran in a wheelchair and on oxygen. He didn't have many teeth but his smile lit up the city of Durham. Normally, I'm like the queen of Christmas. My house looks like Santa's southern home. I LOVE this time of year. I once decorated a friend's house for a Christmas party. People asked who decorated and, well, one thing led to another. Soon I was decorating peoples' homes on the side for extra money. It was creative and a ton of fun!

It was the holiday season and I should've been elated. This season, though, was empty of spirit. I was empty of spirit. I managed to keep a smile on my face, but I felt very vacant, void. I was also way too thin. I was nowhere near the magic, the emotion, the vibration of it, and I couldn't even feel or imagine the essence of Christmas or the holiday season. I felt separate from everything, especially separate from myself. It was a very hollow feeling.

By that point, I was destroyed. No one understood or seemed to care about my pain. The one tablet of Gabapentin was not working, so the doctor upped it to two. That worked for a while as well, but not 100% and not for long. And I was still in a lot of low back and hip pain. This was NOT NORMAL!

By December of 2015, I had lost a lot of weight and felt weak. I could not exercise at all. My ability to use deliberate positive thinking had completely vanished, and I continued to live in a constant state of fear. I wrote the following in my journal on 12/6/15:

> Went to gym today, more to socialize than anything. I am afraid to lift weights (causes spasms in upper and thoracic area), afraid to get on the bike (low back), afraid to get on the elliptical (dizziness), afraid to WALK for fear the pain will increase and intensify. This is nuts. I was in TOP shape a couple of years ago. I have lost 15lbs and feel weak. I am afraid of the atrophy. I just want to be Lynn. I just want to be HEALTHY!!!! I have forgotten how to be happy.

I was utterly shattered, traumatized, horrified, lost. I was miserable in my career. I had been focusing so much attention on trying to get myself well that I had forgotten along the way about my lack of ability to do my job to the level I needed. I somehow forgot about getting back up to speed with the fundamentals of the job. And I guess that, over time, I just accepted that this would be my new baseline. I was in pain every day. Serious, debilitating pain. I tried my very best to keep a smile on my face, and to not let anyone know the extent of my suffering. But the pain kept winning. I had been to ten or eleven specialists, and had several epidurals and a nerve conduction test. Doctors were finding nothing, but were happy to prescribe anti-depressants, opioids, and other drugs. One doctor advised me, "You're just not emotionally ready to admit that you'll have limitations in life." Damn straight, I'm not! It was beyond ridiculous. I felt entirely helpless and was sinking further into despair. I was telling myself, "Enough! I can't do this!" But with each disappointment, dead end, insult, I was somehow able to dig in harder, undertake a new approach to hopefully uncovering answers.

On December 17, 2015, I woke up with severe pain in the left arm. The pain was so intense, I could not use my left arm for several hours. I had another epidural scheduled for 2 p.m. at the pain management center. At about 10:00 a.m., my right hand began to spasm and freeze up. My fingers curled a bit and I could not move my hand. Around noon, my left hand began to freeze as well. I got in my car to head over to my appointment and both hands were frozen—I couldn't move either hand, nor any of my fingers. I was forced to drive to the appointment using the ball of my hands, my wrists and forearms.

My calf pain was awful, unimaginable, and I often dropped to the floor and lost my breath when it hit. I expressed my concern to my primary care doctor AGAIN, reminding her, "I first mentioned this two weeks after the injury. That was eighteen months ago!" "I know, I know," she replied. *That's it? That's all you got?* I was SO beyond frustrated. Luckily, I had two appointments with spine surgeons coming up, one with someone I really liked a lot, Dr. Mathur. He seemed very cautious about surgery, viewing it only as a last resort. He was genuine and spoke with me rather than talking at me. I was learning that bedside manner in my particular situation was highly important to me. Dr. Mathur indicated that although he wasn't yet sure that I would need surgery, all things pointed to that as a strategy.

Mid-January, 2016, the leg pain was intensifying, which I didn't know was even possible. By this time, Dr. Mathur was convinced that a fusion at L4 and L5 would be necessary, and possibly at L5/S1, but he wasn't convinced of the latter yet, just the former. This would involve screws, rods and pins. *OMG! Is this really happening? I thought, This is serious. How on earth will I manage on my own? Who will take care of Buddy? I am terrified. I'll miss a lot of work again. I can't take more bills. But I don't want to wait until my sixties either.* After the visit, I walked slowly out of the building and sat on the bench outside the entrance. I sobbed and sobbed. *How will I afford this? How will I be able to keep my job? I am so afraid.* And then the other voice, the strong voice, that apparently was still in there, came: *I will NOT let fear destroy me!*

By this time, though, I was at a new low. I'd had five epidurals since December and was in constant pain—incredible, agonizing, incomprehensible pain. At this point, I couldn't even go for a walk without pain. I couldn't drive. I couldn't work out. I couldn't vacuum. I couldn't sit. I couldn't sleep. I couldn't stand for too long. I'd dropped twenty pounds, I was only at 15% of my capacity. Maybe less.

I also started experiencing increased sciatica pain in both legs, but more intensely on the left. My doctor upped the Gabapentin again. I had gone from one to two tablets already, and the recommended dosages were up to three tablets a day. So, in order to address this unrelenting pain, the doctor thought it was a good idea to up the dose, especially since it was within dosage guidelines.

Bad idea. Very bad idea.

I became suicidal. I could not live in the pain. I was tired of it. Tired of being on my own. Tired of pills. Tired of everything. Sad beyond belief. Weak beyond recognition. Mentally depleted. I was a wounded animal waiting to die. Lynn was no longer in me. She was nowhere to be found. I just wanted it all to end. My friend, Jamie, in New York got a text from me late at night saying I had a bottle of pills and was going to take them and drink some wine. I couldn't do it anymore. Jamie contacted my friend Reilly, who tried calling, and came over and knocked on my door. But I wouldn't answer the phone. I wouldn't answer the door. I was done. It was over.

CHAPTER EIGHT

SOMETHING'S MISSING (I think it's ME)

*"It is in your moments of decision
that your destiny is shaped."*
-Tony Robbins

The next morning was something of a turning point. My spirit was shouting, "Suicide?! No!! That's not who you are! That makes no sense! There is another way!" I checked the medication side effects and there it was: "These capsules can cause serious side effects, including suicidal thoughts or actions, thoughts about suicide or dying, attempts to commit suicide, new or worsening depression, new or worsening anxiety, panic attacks," and on it went with a laundry list of potentially severe side effects. At that point, a very clear message appeared in my mind: I wanted and needed to make a change. I wanted to be happy. I wanted to catapult myself into health and happiness. I was going for it, whatever "it" meant. I was tired of not fully being me and I desperately wanted to feel whole, vibrant, like the spirit I know I came here to express. Through my life experiences, it seemed I had continued to be pulled further away from the essence of "me." Those last eighteen months had almost fully severed my ties with that essence, and the thought of further separation and of losing my spirit altogether frightened and struck a chord in me.

At a very young age, I was, on some level, afraid to grow apart from the "me" I had come to create and know. I think I was already beginning to recognize the tugging of this physical being away from the essence of the non-physical spirit. When I was about seven years old, I would lay awake at night and wonder what happens to our mind after we die. I didn't understand that I was thinking about consciousness, that word was not yet part of my vocabulary, but it both fascinated and frightened me at the same time. At that age, I viewed body and spirit as very separate, or becoming separate, yet striving to be one. But was there really a separation? I continually contemplated these types of thoughts, questions.

I was born in 1964 and loved the hippy era—the sixties and seventies, The Mamas and the Papas, the bohemia of the day, the styles, everything about it. Well, almost everything. I hated the news stories about conflict, combat, and the starving children in Bangladesh and other areas. At one point, I signed up with UNICEF and corresponded with a young girl named Rajama. I was an idealist, believed in peace, and wanted everyone to love and rejoice in each other. The world was very much with me at a young age. There always seemed to be such a contradiction in what young people were taught and how the world actually was—how we actually treated each other. To me, if we could preach something, then we must know what that looks and feels like and how to demonstrate it. So then, why did it not actually play out that way? I also often pondered why I was born into the country, the town, and the family that I was.

My second grade teacher was Ms. Tesick. She was like a younger version of Carol Brady. She was cute and all the kids' fathers liked to flirt with her. One day, we were talking about the recent news stories of starving children. She asked if any of us thought that could as easily be us. I raised my hand. I was the only one. My parents got a call later that day. I assume now that she may have been concerned about me, maybe for my safety based on my response to her question. But what I was thinking when I raised my hand was this: why wouldn't I have had just as equal a chance or probability of being born into life in the states as in Africa, Russia, India, China, Spain, Chicago, L.A.? Why here? Why not anywhere else?

Several years later, when I was about fourteen years old, I wrote the following poem:

Syncopated sorrows illustrate the
Unseen story
Long implanted in stubborn souls
Successfully stifled by schooling

To me, this meant that my emotions demonstrated a growing disconnect between me and my source, spirit. This disconnect formed a fear that I held underneath my outwardly appropriate façade—a fear that my identity in this world, even though still so driven by my soul, was being continually molded and conditioned by society, schooling, elders, and so on. I had a fear that I would one day forget who I was and that fear, I think, may be exactly what allowed me to stay at least somewhat connected, or at least committed to, that source spirit throughout my life.

So many of us are searching for something in our life. Often, many of us walk around with a little pit in our stomachs, our throats or chest, that feels like something is not 100%, like we are walking through life a bit dull and separate from our true selves. It's as if we intuitively know something is off, and our body is sending us information telling us such. We feel like we are not being who we are supposed to be, not living our life with true purpose as we would like. We often feel stuck, or like we're going through the motions, like a rat on a wheel, but we don't know how to get unstuck, we don't know how to slow down the wheel and jump off, and we don't know how to close the gap between who we truly are and how we outwardly express ourselves through personality.

When I was thirteen, I wrote the following poem, called *World Worth*:

Intense awareness,
hearing, seeing all,
while realizing nothing.
Feeling everything,
while never being touched,
afraid to,
(afraid too.)
Intense awareness,
Monstrous trivialities,
precise moments of
understanding in a world of
deep and endless thought,
snapped out of it to forget its
reasoning.
Afraid this is awareness.
Afraid that it is not.

This poem had a lot to do with detachment and lack of meaning, going through the motions of life without any awareness of who we truly are, incapable of connecting with that self. That's how I feel so many of us go through life: completely unaware, thinking we are aware, when we couldn't be further from awareness. We are feeling beings, but so often, we can feel a myriad of emotions while lacking the ability to connect with the essence, the emotion that comes from fully and intimately knowing our true self. This scared me a little as a young woman as I felt detached from my true self and, in a sense, powerless because of the detachment.

From a very young age, I knew that this was not how I wanted to live. Personally, I wanted more than to go through the motions without any self-realization. I may not have known consciously or specifically what that meant, but intuitively, I knew that I wanted to be self-aware, self-realized (discovering and knowing my true self) and self-actualized (bringing my own uniqueness into the world). Awareness was extraordinarily important to me, even at this early time in my life, possibly because, on some level, I knew I was becoming less aware, and the less aware I became, the more disconnected I felt. I often had moments of precise understanding before suddenly snapping out of it to forget its reasoning, its meaning. I was terrified that this experience was all that awareness was, but also afraid that if this wasn't awareness, that I was in real trouble.

So, in knowing what I did not want, how I did not want to live, I started to slowly develop a general sense for what I did want, how I did want to experience life, but the specifics eluded me. I knew from a young age that I wanted to help people, but I would not know until much older how that would ever take shape.

My mother used to tell this story about me when I was about four years old: We were all getting ready to go to church. My mother summoned me from my bedroom upstairs. I came down, ready to go to mass, but I had a pile of clothes in my arms. She asked me, "What are all those clothes for?" I said, "I'm bringing them to church. They are for Jesus." "For Jesus? Why?" she asked. "Because Jesus has no clothes. He needs to have some, and I want to help him," I responded. You see, each Sunday at mass, I would see the variety of paintings of Jesus that lined the church's interior walls, each painting perfectly placed between an assortment of uniquely distinctive stained glass windows. In every single portrait, Jesus was nearly naked. This made me feel sad and I wanted to help.

After momentarily flirting with suicide, a switch turned on in my mind, and I made a decision. Though still uncertain of the specifics, I made a clear and final decision that major change must and would take place. As I have learned, the first step in making a change is simply the act of deciding to make a change to create our new future. We make a conscious choice to be happy, to reclaim our birthright of bliss, to follow that dream we had, to follow that passion we never followed, leave the job that leaves us unfulfilled, or whatever it is. But we **make** that decision. Practicing positive thoughts and feelings after the TBI was a conscious decision—a simple, easy decision with a simple goal: healing and happiness. This decision, though, was so much more about just my healing and feeling happy. This decision was more about, all about, who Lynn wanted to be and how to create that new reality for myself. And the level of my intention directly matched the level of intensity about that decision. I was tired of living in this reality of pain. I was over it. I wanted myself back—my entire, full, vibrant, creative, deserving and loving self.

Now, in the wake of my suicidal thoughts, I was fully committed to finding Lynn again. I made a clear, strong and unwavering decision to step back into the very best, self-actualized version of me. The decision alone seemed to give me power. By simply identifying the change we want to make, we turn on the creative centers in our brain, and the frontal lobe of our brain starts to look out over the landscape of all other lobes, like a real estate developer looking over beautiful acreage. This is significant, because when your body receives a message from the brain, your body has no idea whether or not the change has happened. Your body has no way of discerning whether the feeling it is experiencing was caused by an actual event or by complete fabrication in the mind. So just by thinking that the change is happening, you give your body a taste of the future potential and you begin that process of shifting. This is why visualization techniques work so well.

In the dawn after my dark night, my decision toward change was so powerful that I was immediately propelled into action. I have NO idea where I found the strength and clarity of mind, but I did. I immediately did two things: 1) I cut back on the meds and prayed with all my heart that the pain would not worsen, and 2) I urged, implored, begged Dr. Mathur to see me. Dr. Mathur immediately ordered an MRI of my lumbar spine. Finally, FINALLY someone ordered an MRI of my low back! And there it was. The hyper-shifting at L4 and L5 that was causing my back pain, and now, per the MRI, a synovial cyst on my spinal cord, which was the culprit behind the electrical calf pain. I definitely needed surgery, and the sooner, the better. Dr. Mathur could see the pain in my eyes and body, and he recognized that I was suffering horribly. The surgery was scheduled for Tuesday, March 1, 2016. In the meantime, I got a second and third opinion, and they both agreed with Dr. Mathur's assessment. I now was excited. I had hope. And on March 1st, I had a fusion and laminectomy, and the cyst was successfully removed from my spinal cord.

Flash back to 2013, when I was looking for a new chiropractor. I found one online and reviewed his website. His office offered a number of services and modalities that were reminiscent of the doctors I used to see in California, and I was intrigued. I had spent a number of years out West, in both southern and northern California, and I missed it dearly. I missed the lifestyle—wellness was simply a part of peoples' lives, as opposed to other regions, where it is more of a choice or a chore. Doctors' approaches out West were always more holistic in view, at least the doctors I saw. As part of his protocol, this chiropractor ordered full spine x-rays. My spine looked great. This was significant, as it clearly showed that, previous to the injury, my spine was absolutely fine. Eighteen long and torturous months later, I finally had answers!

I did it! I persevered through, and someone would now help me out of this hell!

The sun rose in a new way from that day on, and I rose with it.

IMPACT IMPERATIVE #2
CONTINUAL LEARNING

Learning is so important in supporting your transformation. If you were to continue along, day by day, not learning anything new, your brain would continue to fire the same way, and no change would take effect. By simply doing the exercises and following the road map in this book, you will be learning and rewiring your brain. You will develop new neural synaptic connections each time you learn something new. You can boost this impact, though, in any number of ways that represent supportive learning. For example, find teachers, industry experts on the subject, and listen to them on your way to work, or at lunch, or while on the treadmill at the gym. Listen to motivational speakers. Spark up a conversation with someone and really make an effort to learn about them. Create your own exercises that help you along with the process. Just make sure you are continually learning in a way that supports your transformation.

CHAPTER NINE

ROAD TO RECOVERY (Are we there yet?)

"I am not afraid of storms,
for I am learning how to sail my ship."
-Louisa May Alcott

I remained at WakeMed hospital for five days after surgery. The doctors and nurses were wonderful. My surgeon said his jaw dropped to the floor when they cut in and saw just how much my spine had shifted. Often times, the x-rays can't see the entire story. He said this was actually a bit of a precarious situation for me, and it was a good thing I had the surgery without delay. I was the youngest on the hospital floor, and I was optimistic that my initial recovery would be quick, so I was told by other patients and physical therapists. I was hopeful!

My sister came down from Connecticut to stay with me for a week. I slept or rested most of the time. She came in on a Saturday for nine days.

On about day five or so, when the variety of drugs and painkillers start to wear off, things got rough, but they sent me home with Oxycodone, Robaxin, Tramadol, Valium, Vicodin, Hydrocodone—I don't even remember them all, there were so many. I just knew I was going to taper as quickly as possible. It's really interesting and a little frightening how many different types of medications, including numerous opioids, I was prescribed in the months before and after my surgery. I brought a huge bag full of prescriptions, many unopened, most unused, to the fire department for disposal.

The initial recovery took about three months, and required I go on short term disability. As much as I disliked that idea, my health came first and I couldn't let it get me down. I had in-home nurses and physical therapy for the first couple of weeks following surgery. It was a comedy of errors. I was in a lot of pain still, and the physical therapist told me that was not normal, that most people were completely pain-free after surgery. Well, that was a sweeping generalization and completely faulty statement. Everyone is different. Our bodies are highly individual mechanisms. I believed in my own body's intelligence to heal, so I let that go. Because I was in such good shape to begin with, the physical therapists thought I was doing incredibly well and released me fairly soon. She did not see the pain on my face, and must have minimized my comments, but I felt it in my body. The in-home nurses were mediocre. One showed up with a very dusty computer. She was typing on her computer before she told me she was going to remove the dressing over the scar. My doctor had specific instructions as to when the dressing could be removed, and we weren't at that point yet. Still, she continued and asked if I had any scissors to help cut some of the dressing. She also asked if I had any gauze. *No, no scissors. No, no gauze. Uh, don't you?* She rummaged around in her hybrid medical bag-purse. Her purse looked as dusty as the computer keyboard—breeding grounds for germs. She then continued to try to apply a new dressing. "Uh, wait a minute! Can you please wash your hands?" I demanded. I quickly called and requested a new nurse.

It would take about six weeks before I could walk my dog again. I would be able to drive after two or three weeks, but I wasn't in a rush. I wasn't in a rush to drive. I wasn't in a rush to walk. I wasn't in any rush to do anything. I had been through so much the last two years. I wanted to, and deserved to, take my time, go at exactly my own pace, and no one else's. I was very much looking forward to this new chapter. And I was proud of myself for persevering, for continuing to seek answers.

After a couple of weeks, I was sent to physical therapy at the spine center to strengthen my core. I went a few times a week, but they released me quickly, saying I was doing better than most. *Uh, yeah, because I'm twenty years younger than anyone else here, and I'm healthier and more fit than most, but I know my body! I'm nowhere near where I should be,* I thought. Over the next several months, I sought out a couple different physical therapists who were exemplary and committed to getting me back on track. I was an athlete my entire life and physical activity will always be a significant part of my life and self-care program. I had been living with this hyper-shifting in my low back, and now, it was secured, locked in place with hardware. I knew that the fusion at L4 and L5 was going to now put more load on L3 and L5/S1, and I needed to understand how that would impact my exercise program. I was committed to my care and was going to do whatever I needed to do to stay well.

The pain after surgery was draining. I was tired of people telling me, "Oh, yeah, that's just like when I had my rotator cuff surgery," or, "Yeah, that's like when I had surgery on my finger." NO! NO, it is not! It is nothing like that! I appreciated my friends and family who would just listen and let me talk about my experience. That's all I needed. Someone to listen and maybe even crack a joke. Humor always goes a long way in my book.

After some recovery, I was able to walk again! I enjoyed walking, and had such nice memories of my walks before the chaos of pain. I found that I could once again draw upon those memories and revive and relive the emotions I used to feel. I had spent that time thinking good feeling thoughts, being appreciative, and I delighted in listening to and learning from my mentors. Like running used to, walking now helped release my stress and inspire creativity. I looked forward to reconnecting to that experience. Suddenly, my world was becoming brighter. In fact, the color of grass, of flowers, of the leaves on the trees were all so much brighter! I felt I was on my way back to life. Back to Lynn.

I had worked my way up to a half-hour of walking, and eventually, an hour or more per day. I had new pain now, though. My lower right back was constantly in pain, but a more dull, although intense, pain. I assumed it would work itself out. After all, I had just invited steel rods and screws to live inside me and this was incredibly foreign to my body. Perhaps it was partly muscular. I was not about to worry about it. Dr. Mathur had given me a new lease on life and I was OVER THE MOON!

I immediately got back on track with my mindset practice. I began listening to my mentors and found new ones. I listened while walking, while in the car—any and every opportunity I could. I practiced what my teachers were offering. I now felt I had purpose; I had no idea yet what that purpose was, but I knew I was here on earth for a reason. I wanted to become fully self-realized and fully self-actualized, and I was excited to experience that journey. I did not want to take the past with me into my future. That period was over and it didn't exist any longer. The only thing that I would take from that chapter was lessons learned, but all the rest - in the dumpster. I was fully looking forward to my future, and although I didn't exactly know what the future held, I certainly knew how it felt: robust, empowering, fulfilling, awesome!

My walks had become a place of creation and imagination, and I never tired of my walking routes. They were quite pleasant, quiet with various peaceful cul-de-sacs, with beautiful homes, garnished with nicely maintained lawns. The topography was fairly flat, but the picturesque neighborhood did incorporate a few hills as well. Bonus! I love walking hills. That wasn't always the case.

When I moved from Irvine, California up to San Francisco, a runner and former cyclist at the time, I had experience with some hills from time to time. But in San Francisco, hills were everywhere! It was hills on steroids. They were inevitable. A part of life. A given, like taxes. There was no getting around them. Period. I hated the idea of running hills all the time, but over time, I came to fall in love and even crave them. There was something about the recovery, too. I could bring my heartrate down in just a few seconds and I was ready for another hill.

I lived in a flat on Lake Street, in the inner Richmond area of San Francisco. I could see the Golden Gate Bridge from my window, and the Presidio was adjacent. I would run to Ocean Beach and then back through Lincoln Park and Seacliff, past my place, then through the Presidio, Marina, back through Richmond and home. I ran between seven to thirteen miles each day. I loved it! I sought out hills wherever I traveled.

Travel had always been a large part of my career, both national and international, and I was highly adept at scouting out the local gyms or the hotels that had a fitness center. If there were no gyms or fitness center (often times, where I traveled, there weren't), I would stash exercise bands in my bag for some core work in my hotel room. I would always evaluate the neighborhood ahead of time so that I could devise a running route. Running hills in San Francisco made me strong and fast. Soon, my leisurely recreational eight-minute mile pace would improve to 7:20, then seven-minute miles. That was good for me. I was good with it. Super proud of myself.

My recovery had thus far been a little like running the San Francisco hills: torturous on the uphill, and trying to enjoy the downhill as much and for as long as possible. But now, I will walk. Not run. And I'm beyond okay with that, too. The only thing I'm focused on now is the journey into my future, whatever that holds.

EXERCISE:

- Find mentors, teachers, industry leaders, and listen or read on a routine basis. Learn as much as you can and have fun with it! Continue with the previous exercises and journal.

PART II
The Learning of a New Self

CHAPTER TEN

STOP BELIEVING THE STORY YOU'RE TELLING YOURSELF! (It's bullshit.)

"The only limits you have are the limits you believe."
-Wayne Dyer

I finally returned full time to work in June of 2016. I was so excited to be back and part of a team again. People at the bank were kind and extended their sincere sorrow for what I had been enduring the past couple of years. A few shared their own stories of horrific injuries they or their loved ones had endured as a way of conveying to me that they understood the pain and hardship. Some of these stories were incredible and I was honored that my co-workers shared their experiences with me.

Shortly after my return, I saw an email regarding a three-day leadership retreat. It always intrigues and puzzles me when I see such announcements, and raises a number of questions in my mind: How do you expect to create a team of leaders in three days? How will a three-day retreat lead to any substantial and sustainable changes, especially with the same old tired agenda in place? How are you going to break and evolve the old culture and habits of the team and organization in three days? Exactly what do you hope to accomplish by this, other than spending a lot of time and resources on a three-day pep rally? Companies spend billions on such trainings and retreats each year with little lasting impact. I just always found these events to be a huge waste of resources. Of course, these getaways are very well intended and often a good pick-me-up boost to morale (and goodness knows, it was needed at the time), but it's usually quite temporary, and very rarely, if ever, successful in creating overnight leaders or lasting change. I was finding in my own evolution that sustainable change takes more than a few good dinners, drinks, speeches and awards. It takes a lot of looking within, digging deep, internal discovery and accessing the subconscious, where habits reside and where real change takes place. Folks returned from the retreat, and everything was back to normal within about eight hours.

I was walking an hour or more at a time each day by July, 2016. Sometimes, time permitting, I'd indulge in more than one walk. I continued to go to physical therapy and was also incorporating some gym time and routine massage. My low back pain persisted. It was not getting any better, and now both feet hurt from time to time. Still, I continued along, resolved to get to the bottom of this new pain, determined that I would not let it run or ruin my life.

It was right around this time that I began lamenting how unhappy I was with my job. Now, to many, I was, ostensibly, very successful. I had a good paying job, an established career that allowed me to develop a unique variety of skills, and I'd built upon a wide range of professional roles and experience as well as a number of environments and cultures. But I did not feel successful. I felt unfulfilled, less than, and stagnant. It bothered me that I was so absolutely miserable in my career. It really didn't make a lot of sense as to why I was so happy in every other aspect of my life. These areas were not perfect by a long shot. For example, I had no significant romantic relationship in my life, but I was content. I hadn't yet developed a lot of friends and supportive relationships, but I was working on it and was content. My physical health wasn't where I wanted it to be, but I was appreciative to have come so far, so I was okay with that too. Yet, I was so dissatisfied in my career.

I started to wonder what kind of thoughts I have about work, what kind of story I may be telling myself about work that is holding me back from enjoying myself in that environment. Even if my job's not perfect, surely I can still find some contentment in it, just as I have in the other not-so-perfect areas of my life. I developed this little exercise, "Fill in the Blank." I wrote down Work is _____. Then I began to fill in the blanks. I wrote: Work is hard. Work is a grind. Work is stressful. Work is political. Work is exhausting. Work is intense. I had developed a really negative narrative.

I had created a belief system around work that was not serving me well. I was holding an incredible amount of resistance toward my work, and my emotions were letting me know this on a daily basis. I was going headstrong upstream. I actually had strong somatic responses when I thought about work. One thing I learned is that whenever there is a highly emotional or somatic response to something, it's very important to check in with that experience, because that is directly where our thoughts and energy are going, and our body and emotions are letting us know, "Hey! This is really important stuff, and it's making me feel BAD, so you need to look into this!"

I decided to shift and try to write a better story. I wrote "Work is challenging." Not exactly a 100% turn upstream, but a shift. I continued to write: Work is flexible. Work pays well. I started writing things like: I work with an amazing group of collaborative and supportive colleagues. My boss is awesome and does not micro-manage. I have a flexible schedule. And on and on. Simply put, I began to focus on all of the positive aspects of my career. At the same time, I practiced unconditional living on a daily basis for ME, not taking any actions at all based on what others thought I should do or say. I began trying to re-write my story (belief) about work as part of my routine of daily exercises. It would later prove to be highly transformational.

That simple exercise got me thinking: If I had created a story and belief about my work, what other beliefs about other aspects of my life, or just about me in general, am I telling myself? This made me dig even deeper to try to gain awareness of not only my limiting thoughts, but the *beliefs* that had been formed in me. I was taken back to a memory from fourth grade. I was in a sprint race during a field day at school, and the girl I was racing against fell and hit the ground really hard. Stunned by the thump of her body hitting the ground, my impulse was to stop and see if she was okay. I went over to help her, but was halted by the sound of a hoard of parents screaming at me to keep running. No one was helping this girl who was clearly injured by her fall. They seemed more interested in seeing me finish and win the race than in lending any assistance to the poor girl. That was a really tough lesson for me about our society! I know it sounds silly now, but looking back, I no doubt formed a belief at that moment that people do not care for each other. I had definitely carried this belief throughout my life. I never relied on people for my wellbeing, because, on some level, I didn't think people cared or at least weren't interested in offering care. That was, in part, why it was difficult for me to reach out to ask for help in the days, weeks, and months (years, in fact) following the injury.

So, just like in the "Fill in the Blank" exercise, where there was actually a good story I could tell about my work, clearly there must be a positive to this. My belief that people don't care for or help each other only represented one side of the coin. Perhaps, on the other side of the coin was the fact that I wanted to help people, and if I have that desire, I thought, then surely there are many others who do as well. Clearly, the belief wasn't even true. Of course, there are people who love to help others! Of course, there will be some that prefer not to, and that's okay! This belief was now no longer part of my make-up. Belief debunked. This again, was a really simple tool, but it was proving to be incredibly powerful, empowering.

This exercise prompted me to really understand even more fully that I—we all—hold a lot of limiting beliefs. Beliefs are simply thoughts that are repeated over time. Limiting beliefs are beliefs that constrain us or hold us back. They are negative in nature and are usually based in fear or lack. For example, "I don't have enough money" is a belief based in lack. "I'm not loved" is a belief based in fear of rejection. We all have thousands of thoughts running through our heads each day that tell us negative messages throughout the day, such as "I'm not smart enough," or, "I'm not worthy of that," or, "I can't do it," "There's something wrong with me," or, "I might take my shirt off in public!"

According to experts, such as Bruce Lipton, Dr. Joe Dispenza and Joe Vitale, among others, most of these thoughts are initially formed in our first six to seven years of life, and become fairly solidified into our behaviors and personalities by the time we are thirty-five years old. Of course, some thoughts and beliefs continue to be formed as we go through life, but most are formed in our earliest years. So, over time, we develop a mind-made version of our self, of who we think we are, based on the thoughts and beliefs we've formed.

As a simple example, when I was in second grade, I did poorly on a reading comprehension quiz. Heretofore, I had done very well, and was ahead of kids my age in reading, and all other subjects, for that matter. But now, I was having trouble, and I felt bad. I felt stupid. I don't remember much more than that, but chances are that the thought of being stupid could have, over time, formed the belief in me that "I'm not smart enough." (This one has haunted me throughout my life!)

Some thoughts and beliefs result from trauma. For example, when

I was fifteen years old, a tornado unexpectedly formed in my hometown and was aimed directly at my house. I was alone in my bedroom at the time, talking with a friend on the phone. I was laying on my back on the bed, my head turned toward the window, looking at the tree outside. The weather was humid but otherwise calm. Then, things changed instantly. I heard the roar of the wind barreling down the street, uprooting the first tree that would fall on the house, the top branch thrusting through my bedroom window, landing within inches of me, raising sheer panic in my mind and body. I immediately went into fight or flight mode and started to run down the stairs and (not thinking) toward the front door. When I frantically opened the front door, a second tree uprooted and came crashing down right in front of me, again, missing me by inches. Terrified, and having never been in a tornado before, I tried to have the presence of mind to remember what people are supposed to do in a tornado. I made a run for it to the neighbor's house and, without notice or knocking, swung open the door to find them sitting and chatting over tea, completely unaware that a tornado had just hit. Though I was fine physically, fear had made an imprint on my brain. For years and years, strong winds absolutely terrified me, and I felt unsafe and in danger in any storm situation following that event. In this example, there was a traumatic event that triggered specific thoughts, feelings and emotions that my brain recorded as a memory. The memory of the tornado produced highly elevated feelings and emotions of fear due to the traumatic nature of the event. It was far easier for me to recall this experience than, say, me doing poorly on a reading comprehension test.

After deconstructing and shifting my beliefs about work and people being uncaring, I began to identify and shift even more limiting beliefs. The first thing I did whenever one came up was to ask if it's even true. I called this exercise "Truth or Lies." After identifying the belief, I would ask "Is that true? Is it a fact?" For example: "I can't exercise because I don't have time" is not a fact. There is always enough time to exercise, even if in your office or home, but "I don't exercise because I broke my femur" is most probably a fact. Most of the time, our limiting thoughts and beliefs are not true at all, but are instead based on false perceptions that we generated back when we were very young, that we've just repeated over the years. What I was coming to learn was that most of the limiting beliefs we hold aren't factual at all! LIES! Complete BS! So, we've been holding on to thousands (yes, thousands) of limiting, false, untrue beliefs that work directly in opposition to our true self's full potential. This is extraordinary! It's astonishing because it means that we have bought into, we have come to believe, a false narrative about who we are and what we are capable of. I would continue to contemplate this as my practice progressed.

My walks were becoming inspiring, fun and blissful beyond description. I routinely practiced "My Favorite Things," thinking of my favorite best feeling thought and imagining new best feeling thoughts. It was so much fun. I was also teaching myself all kinds of new exercises. I began revisiting the concepts of the law of attraction fairly religiously. Never would I say to myself, "Go away, this thought that I don't want," as this is still focusing on the bad thought. Rather, I'd simply acknowledge the thought and replace it with something better. Stated differently, instead of focusing on what I didn't want to think about, I focused on what I did want to think about, and reached for the matching heartening emotion. My goal was to bring the emotion to the same level, in alignment with, the thought. In other words, I placed intention behind my thoughts and this produced an even more amplified emotion.

Sometimes we can think a thought, but if we don't feel a corresponding emotion, we then lack motivation or belief in the thought itself. In other words, you can have positive thoughts or say positive affirmations all day long, but if you lack a matching emotion, it won't get you very far. In those cases where I had trouble matching the emotion or getting to a best feeling thought, I'd simply slow down and try to at least shift the thought into a more positive direction where a matching emotion could be found.

I looked forward to my walking time every day very much. I mention it numerous times because the exercise routine felt that significant to me, it brought such simple delight. My pain continued to persist, but I was not focused on it. I was focused only on my amazing future. Now, I knew I couldn't immediately create an amazing brand new shiny future overnight. I knew it would be a shift, but the process itself was becoming so fun, so enjoyable, I was 100% down for the ride, no matter the time it took. In fact, the longer, the better, because the process of this evolution was so enjoyable. Further, I did not require anything to manifest in form immediately. My elevated emotions and feelings of joy were manifestations in themselves.

EXERCISES:

- Do the "Fill in the Blank" exercise. Pick a topic—work, exercise, home cooking, healthy eating—and see what you come up with.
- Can you think of a defining moment in which you began to form a limiting belief in your life?

IMPACT IMPERATIVE #3
ELEVATED EMOTIONS

It is not enough to simply practice positive thoughts and phrases. To really make change, our new thoughts must be paired with higher, elevated emotions. You must be able to feel the thoughts, feel the vision, emote the feelings. Great change is never achieved in a state of contraction, hate, anger, or any of those lower vibration states. Great things are achieved when we are in a state of expansion, love, appreciation, grace, those higher, elevated vibration states. When you combine your intention with an elevated emotion, you will feel it in your body. Your body begins to experience the future vision you are creating in your mind, even if it isn't yet manifest. When this happens, great change has already begun and great things will happen.

CHAPTER ELEVEN

OOH, THE POSSIBILITIES!
(Can you see and feel them?)

"When nothing is sure, everything is possible."
-Margaret Drabble

In late September, 2016, work took me to a small town about an hour south. It was a lovely sunny, warm day, perfected by a bright blue North Carolina sky. By now, I had become accustomed to driving a variety of sleepy rural country roads and, on this particular morning, I was inspired to try following a brand new country route. I was about five miles from my destination. A field of cows grazing was to my left, and to my right, a beautiful still lake adjacent to a cornfield with corn ripe for harvest, when suddenly a wave of absolute euphoric JOY washed over me. I was literally stunned. So stunned, in fact, that I needed to pull over to the side of the road. I couldn't recall ever feeling this type of intense bliss ever before. It was quite a foreign feeling. It was so unfamiliar, even uncomfortable, yet, at the same time, it felt very natural. I was perplexed by the incongruity of the paired feelings—the natural, blissful joy meeting the unfamiliar and uncomfortable. Something told me that I simply needed to stay with this joy, this bliss, to fully enjoy it and, more importantly, to rehearse it until I could recall it in an instant. This feeling fully and absolutely commanded my attention. This was such a strikingly powerful emotion that I needed to record it as permanently as possible in my brain, body and memory. I stayed with this feeling as long as I could. The awkwardness ultimately dissolved and the joy remained. The feeling was SO incredible. My eyes welled, and I thanked God for this person I was becoming and the feelings of joy and bliss that I was increasingly and fairly consistently experiencing. I thought, *I'm not at all the same person I was a year ago or two years ago. I can't wait to see who I'll be in another year!* It was as if my entire identity, my personality was shifting, and my experience of the world was shifting with it. The lens through which I was viewing my world was illuminating, and my experience was consequently far brighter, more interesting, and highly satisfying.

Now proficient in recognizing negative thoughts that create negative emotions, I was quite curious to uncover what positive thoughts I had been thinking to create this amazing feeling. I wasn't sure. I couldn't uncover a specific thought or action that brought on this wave of beautiful bliss, but it didn't matter. What mattered now was that I had felt it and let it soothe me, and I found a way to instantly recall the feeling again. It was an amazing gift.

By now, I was listening incessantly to my mentors, and was finding new ones. I listened in the car to and from work, driving to the coffee shop, driving to meetings, while running errands. I listened while out walking, walking my dog, while stretching or just hanging out at home— any opportunity that presented itself. Over time, it was an amazing feeling. I began to feel more and more empowered. Robust. Confident. Closer to Lynn. Nothing and no one could bother me.

Eventually, with all of my learning, repetition, emoting, appreciation and practice, I was reaching a state of continual bliss. And there was my answer! Of course! It was one thing to practice good thoughts and feelings, but the incredible joyful event that I had just experienced was the result of *much, much more* than that! That feeling washed over me like a homecoming, and I knew it would be lasting, sustainable. It was now part of me, part of my circuitry, and that only happened because of my practice of awareness, continued learning, elevated emotions, appreciation, repetition and discipline—what I would later collectively refer to as the Six Impact Imperatives. During my journey, I came to understand that these were essential and absolute requisites for success in this process.

I suddenly realized that, until now, I had been walking through life with a serious deficit of joy. But after that experience, I would never go back to living that way—living like my former self.

I think this was actually the first time that I began to believe, no, to know, that the pain was really truly behind me. But more than that, my entire future lay ahead of me, and I had the power to shape and mold and play with that future. I had never thought this was possible before, not consciously with such conviction anyway. I was so excited about the future, even though I had no idea what it would hold. The past was the past and I could freely let it, with all its pain, melt into nothingness. What an amazing and empowering feeling! I simply became excited considering the possibilities.

The world of quantum physics is all about possibility thinking, so over the years, with my transformation in mind, I've developed a strong interest in this model. I've come to understand that my ability to imagine different possibilities lays in my genetic make-up, in my connection to the universe, and is nearly a direct reflection of quantum physics. Just as the universe creates dimensions of possibilities, so can I imagine the possibilities of my future and of my potential.

There are two distinctive models of physics: the Newtonian (old) model and the quantum (new) model. I am not a scientist, however, I have found during my personal spiritual journey that an understanding of these models (especially the quantum model) has been essential to my personal understanding, perspective, and growth. In my own experiences, I've learned several times over that life is definitely not linear. My acceptance of this idea has helped me in times of great challenges to go with and in the flow of the experience.

Most of us have learned the classical, or Newtonian, model of how the world works. This model is based on predictability, logic, matter (which is made up of particles, atoms, and subatomic particles), and mathematics. Under this Newtonian or classical view, things are predictable, or can be predicted. Life is, generally speaking, linear. Our five senses help us to experience or perceive all that exists in reality. If we cannot perceive it, it doesn't exist.

In contrast, the quantum physics model is entirely about energy first and possibility, whether or not it can be perceived in the moment. Life is not linear. We are electromagnetic beings with fluctuating vibrational frequencies that will attract similar vibrations. In the quantum model, just because we cannot perceive something in the material sense does not mean it doesn't exist. In the quantum model, there are infinite possibilities, and it is up to each of us to choose what possibilities we want to experience in our existence. The quantum model is all about energy. We are far more than the contents of our minds. We can observe our mind, but we can also create it. The quantum field only responds to who or what you are being, not what you are doing or thinking. Under the quantum model, just because we can't see something, doesn't mean it doesn't exist.

So the question for us is: can we believe in something—a new future, a new outlook, a new mind, more wealth—if it is not yet manifest in the material, physical form? Under the classical model, possibilities that we cannot observe are outside of us; there is a distinct separation between what is (in our perception of the world) and what could be (separate from our reality). But according to the quantum model, there is no separation, and what is far is actually near. The following illustrates the difference:

Common view of possibility thinking:

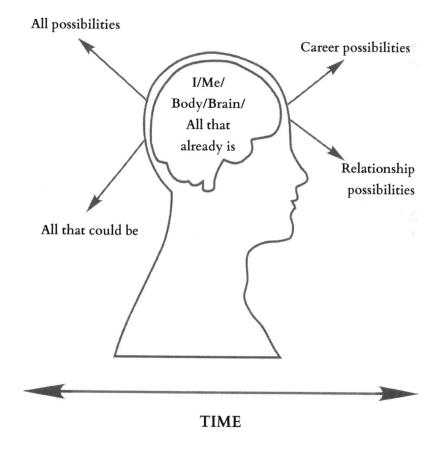

Many of us view possibilities (that car, that job, relationship, or other possibilities) as being outside of ourselves.

Quantum, current view of possibility thinking:

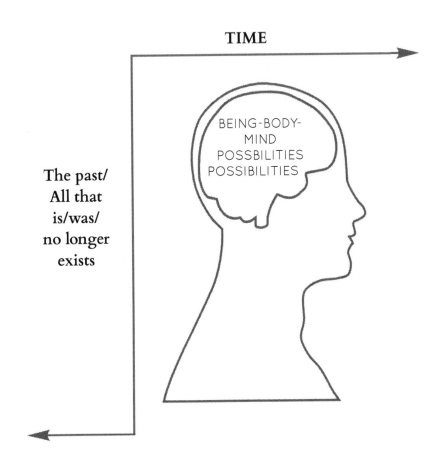

Possibilities lay within each of us. We just need to tap into the infinite possibilities.

So, how does this fit into our discussion on shifting our mindset, our beliefs, thoughts, attitudes and identities? Well, as we know, our brain is constantly and continually influencing our body, and vice versa. There is a strong relationship between mind and body. They are not separate. The body, though, tends to have more influence over the brain due to conditioning over time. Before you even think about reaching for a cup of coffee, neurons in your arm and hand are firing and have already begun the process of reaching for the cup, well in advance of the thought registering in your brain. When you go to brush your teeth in the morning, signals are telling your hand to pick up the toothbrush before your brain thinks about the specific action. Do you tend to grab a drink to relax after a long day at work without even giving it thought? These are all habits formed from constant conditioning.

If we use the quantum model and possibility thinking, we can take control and retrain this body-brain connection so that the body is no longer in control of the mind; the app is no longer running us from the background. We are now choosing how the app will run. We are now determining what our future will hold. We are now involved in possibility thinking and future reality creation.

EXERCISES:

- Take some time to consider your current state of being and your ideal state of being. Is there a gap between the two? We are never really separate from our true self—it's really an illusion. The gap is something of an illusion. What is your vision of the best "you" you can be? If you feel you already are that best version and there is no gap between you and the ideal you, that's great! If you had no limitations in this world, if you had no conditions, if you were free to just be you, what would that look like? How would you express yourself in life? Do you possess talents that are not being actualized? If you were achieving your fullest potential, what would that look like? Can you envision and feel the essence of the new version of your being you wish to create? What are the components of your future essence?

- Now, consider the story you have been telling yourself about who you are now. Is there a difference?

- Compare the traits and stories of the "you" that you "think you are" and the true essence of you, the ideal you, in the following table:

	Old/Current	Future/Ideal
Trait 1	*Shy*	*Confident*
Trait 2	*Limited*	*Creative*
Trait 3	*Fear of failure*	*Empowered*
Lie 1	*I'm not smart*	
Truth 1		*I'm highly intelligent*
Lie 2	*I'm broke*	
Truth 2		*Money is abundant*

IMPACT IMPERATIVE #4
APPRECIATION

Appreciation throughout this process is meaningful for a number of reasons. The state of appreciation is really high up there on the vibration scale. When we are in a state of appreciation, we are in the receptive, allowing mode. In this state of being/mind, we are more creative, and less in our negative thinking. In appreciation, we are placing our attention and, therefore, our energy on things, people, circumstances, and events that are pleasing to us, for which we give thanks. This allows us to step away from our problems and into our solutions. Although gratitude and appreciation are similar, and both have a high vibration, I prefer to use "appreciation." Usually, when someone uses "gratitude," there is still some essence of a problem tied to the past, or something that has been overcome, and it's the related feeling and emotion that is important, so if there is an undertone of anger or fear or any other lower vibration, that will be the energy activated. Appreciation is so much purer in its essence and vibration. When we say things like, "I really appreciate you," or, "I appreciate my career," we are living in the present and not activating emotions of the past. Be cognizant and pay attention to the purity of your sentiment.

CHAPTER TWELVE

ATTITUDE OF ~~GRATITUDE~~ APPRECIATION

"Dwell on the beauty of life. Watch the stars,
and see yourself running with them."
-Marcus Aurelius

By October of 2016, I am not out of pain, but I am experiencing such profound levels of appreciation, and the more I am in that state, the more good things seem to happen, the more beauty I see, the better I feel.

Appreciation is immensely important in this journey, as without it, we cannot transform. The term is often used interchangeably with gratitude. Both terms have been assigned various meanings, often associated with an action of giving thanks or saying thank you. Personally, I prefer the term "appreciation" to "gratitude" only because, very often, when someone expresses gratitude, there is an element of overcoming something negative in the past. Often, when people express "gratitude," there is also a vibration of, a reference to, a past problem. ("I'm so grateful to be out of that relationship.") However, it is, of course, possible to express gratitude without any attachment to the past or any negative undertone.

Real gratitude is an emotion that goes much further and deeper and is essential to our growth and happiness in life. As defined by Harvard Medical School, gratitude is *"a thankful appreciation for what an individual receives, whether tangible or intangible. With gratitude, people acknowledge the goodness in their lives... As a result, gratitude also helps people connect to something larger than themselves as individuals—whether to other people, nature, or a higher power."*

I love this definition because it uses both gratitude and appreciation within it, and the two words seem to share the same energy. This definition also touches upon a few important points: One, what is received need not be tangible. Simply, a heightened emotion is a manifestation for which we can be grateful. Secondly, when we are grateful, appreciative, we recognize all the goodness in our lives, whether big or small, tangible or intangible. And finally, living in and practicing gratitude truly does help us to connect to something greater than ourselves. When we are in a state of appreciation or gratitude, we are in the best possible state of receiving, and that helps us connect to our dreams, our future, others, and our true self as well.

But how do we learn to live, to remain in a state of gratitude and appreciation? Again, it is a practice. For those of us not accustomed to living in this state, it takes a little work. What is the first thing we think about when we awake each day? What is the first emotion we feel? Are we aware of our first breath when we wake? Are we aware of how we feel? What we think? Do we awake and give thanks and gratitude for our existence, or for all the good in our lives? Chances are, the answer is no. I have done numerous surveys with people, asking two things: When you awake each day, what are the first three things you think of and what are the first three things you do? The answers were fairly predictable. 70% of the responses typically included something like the following:

First three thoughts: What am I going to eat? Ugh, work. Who liked my post on Facebook?

First three actions: Look at phone (social media), go to the bathroom, and get a cup of coffee.

Only a limited few responded with thoughts of gratitude or action of envisioning an awesome day ahead. Most people awake with negative thoughts and predictable actions, and that is because we tend to approach each and every day based on the patterns of our past. But if we take this approach, we can't really expect our future to change, can we?

For those of you who observe the Christmas holiday, do you remember the excitement of Christmas as a child? Remember the thrilling anticipation of Christmas Eve, the sheer exuberance waking up Christmas morning and the amazing awe that overcame you as you thought about the surprises of this unforgettable day that was about to unfold?! You had no idea what would be under the tree. All you knew was that you were overflowing with enthusiasm and cheerful wonder about what this incredibly special day would bring. You had absolutely no interest in the past, the bully at school, or the homework that would be due after the break. Your focus was simply and entirely upon the magic of your wonderful life right there in the present day and in the joyous future of what was to come.

So, why don't we awake every morning with the same excitement? Perhaps you are thinking that at five years old, you were completely without the numerous and competing responsibilities of adulthood, so you actually could be free in the moment. But why not try to deliberately set your focus each day upon the positive possibilities for the coming day rather than the pessimistic patterns of the past? This is where appreciation comes into play, because getting to that heightened emotion of pure pleasure about the possibilities requires a certain amount of appreciation.

During my journey to heal my mind and body, I recognized and experienced firsthand the wonderful magic of being in a stated of appreciation, but not simply by saying "I appreciate" something, but by really feeling the essence of that word in my emotions and body. I continued to develop appreciation exercises that I could routinely practice.

I called the first exercise "Doze with Desired Deliberation and Awake with Awareness and Appreciation." I developed this when a deadline for a report was causing me a little stress. The report was due the next day and I still had some work to do, so I was nervous about getting the answers I needed to get the report reviewed and distributed on time. That night, before going to sleep, I deliberately set my intentions for the coming day. Just before falling asleep, I said to myself, "Tomorrow, I will have all the answers I need and the work will flow effortlessly." The next morning, I sat in front of the computer screen and the answers came just as intended: effortlessly, easily, timely and organized. Within an hour, the report was finalized, reviewed, and disseminated.

The next morning, before even thinking about picking up the phone to check social media or text messages, and before even getting out of bed, I simply said to myself, "This is going to be an awesome day!" and *I meant it!* To this day, I do this exercise every morning, making this statement or something similar, and always with intention and emotion. Every morning upon waking, l also now ask myself, "What am I going to create today?"

It's not necessary to define what "awesome" represents in your day. The most important thing is to get into that state of emotion of appreciation for the day to come. Sometimes, I choose to thank God or the universe for bestowing me with this day; the present of this new day which I am about to unwrap. At first, I had to make a note to practice these exercises but, over time, it became second nature, automatic. I now head to slumber excited for the next morning, and awake every day in an amazing mood.

I appreciated my jaunts through my community, adorned with its beautifully landscaped yards and lovely trees. There was a particular road where two trees in the distance seemed to be reaching out to each other, their respective branches extending towards the other as if trying to hold hands from opposite sides of the street. I created the "Walking into My Future" appreciation exercise: When I got to this point in the walk, I would pretend that the space between the trees was my future and, with every stride, I was stepping right into it. Nothing existed behind my back, only my present (for an instant) location and my exciting future, for which I expressed my appreciation, as if it already existed and I was simply about to experience it. I would imagine whatever would ideally be on the other side of the trees.

One of my mentors has been Abraham (Esther) Hicks, which many know from the movies *What the Bleep Do We Know* and *Law of Attraction.* Hicks goes on what is referred to as "rampages of appreciation," where words and phrases of appreciation and gratitude simply flow for minutes on end. It's highly inspiring and uplifting. I devised my own little exercise that I call "Appreciation Alphabet Soup." While out on my walks, I look into the sky and give thanks to the universe, recognizing my place in it, far beyond this temporary physical existence, but also in the physical form. Then I express appreciation with a simple sentence that includes a word of gratitude, first beginning with the letter A, and replacing the word of gratitude with another that begins with the next letter in the alphabet. It is very important that the word is matched with a feeling—a heightened emotion that is connected with each word—because this is how we reprogram our brain circuitry to new patterns, and redesign our mind to new possibilities. Here's how it goes:

Thank you, universe, for all of the beauty and goodness in my life. I am so thankful, for the universe is always appreciating me, bestowing good things, creating with me, developing, empowering me, fulfilling me, guiding me, helping me, inspiring me, joking, knowing, loving, moving, nurturing, opening doors, providing for me, quieting, restoring, supporting, trusting, uncovering, validating, wonderful, xenial, yay (!), and zestful.

I sometimes do this in Spanish just for fun, and I always try to do it more than once, incorporating as many new words as possible.

Not only am I practicing everything I've learned and taught myself, but I'm continuing to learn, continuing to add to my practice, and continuing to be appreciative and inspired! (By this point, I think my positivity might be annoying to some!) I'm now like a dog with its head out the window, just enjoying the ride.

EXERCISE:

- Practice these exercises every day for 7–10 days (or longer). What kinds of shifts do you experience?

CHAPTER THIRTEEN

IT'S THE MOST WONDERFUL TIME OF YEAR

"Success is not the key to happiness.
Happiness is the key to success."
-Albert Schweitzer

In November, 2016, business required me to be in Wilmington, NC. I left on a Sunday and took my time. I traveled along the back roads. It was far more pleasant to drive the North Carolina country roads than Interstate 40, and I wasn't yet comfortable spending too much time on the highway given the dizziness I experienced at higher speeds. I stopped at a gas station and filled up the tank. Before continuing on, I opened YouTube on my phone to find something interesting to listen to, ideally having to do with the mind-body connection. I don't recall the title of the video, but, apparently, I was intrigued enough to hit play. The interviewer introduced his guest, Dr. Joe Dispenza, and Dr. Joe began to tell the story of how he came to where he is in his life.

Dr. Joe was a tri-athlete in his earlier years. When he was twenty-one years old, he was in the cycling portion of a race in Southern California, and when he turned a corner on his bike, an oncoming Mack truck hit and catapulted him forty feet. He was told he would never walk again and that he'd be in a body cast for a year. After putting the body cast on the very first time, he made a pact with himself and said, "If I can walk out of this hospital, I will dedicate the remainder of my life to neuroscience." Twelve weeks later, Joe Dispenza walked out of the hospital. He is now a world-renowned neuroscience researcher, lecturer and educator.

I listened further as Dr. Joe spoke about changing your thinking to change how you feel, and changing your personality to change your personal reality. It was fascinating! He was explaining, in scientific terms, all the things I had been experiencing! This was amazing to me. I couldn't stop listening. I sought out as many of his videos and books as possible, as they were so resonant. I felt so aligned with his teachings, and I still do.

Heretofore, I had no understanding of why my transformation thus far was so successful, but it really didn't matter. I just knew it worked, much like I understand that I can get light by turning on the light switch without understanding electricity. Dr. Joe was now explaining the science behind my light switch! It wasn't just some weird unexplainable phenomenon—there was actual science behind it. I don't know why, but that empowered me, and I wanted more. I wanted more than just this state of joy. I wanted to literally create my new reality, but I wasn't sure yet what that looked like.

After my injury, I learned very quickly that negative stress of any kind was unhealthy and I'd become symptomatic. In the early stages, when a stressor produced a negative thought and response, I learned how to quickly replace with a positive thought and response. This made me and my brain feel better. That much I understood. What I didn't understand, though, was that I was shortening the refractory period to a stress response.

The refractory period is the reaction time to a thought, the period of time immediately following the thought. According to Dr. Joe's teachings, that's when real change takes place. That's also where you begin taking control back from the operating system or application in the background—your negative thinking on autopilot. Your body is no longer in control. You are. That resonated as well because, for the first time in a very long time, I felt like I was finally taking control. He was explaining how we become addicted to our thinking, since every thought we think produces a chemical reaction. Unfortunately, most of the thinking we do is negative, he explained, and therefore, we are literally addicted to our negative thoughts. I wanted to be addicted to positive thoughts!

I was now feeling empowered, thirsty to learn more, and began to expand beyond just thought words, my inner dialogue, to the spoken word. I started listening to how others phrased things and then began to pay attention to my own spoken phrases. My friend, Jamie, was contemplating moving to North Carolina from New York, but she had some fears. "What if it all goes so wrong?" she asked, to which I replied, "What if it all goes so right?" We laughed at the reality that we often think of the possibility of failure before success. Now, before this, I thought I was becoming a beacon of positivity, but when I began to pay attention to how I was speaking in addition to what I was thinking, I found I had some more work to do.

It made a lot of sense, though. The spoken word is just an extension of thoughts and, over time, we develop ways of expressing ourselves that are aligned with our thinking. I started to practice. For example, instead of saying, "Things could be worse," I would say instead, "Things are going pretty good!" I would listen to others' negative speak and would find ways in my mind to shift the language. I asked a friend how she liked a certain movie, and she responded, "It wasn't so bad." The better response would've been, "It was pretty good." Rather than saying, "I'm so broke," state confidently, "I'm overcoming a cash flow issue."

I would also pay attention to how my body felt after a negative thought or reaction. As a simple example that we can probably all understand, does it feel good or bad if we curse at someone in traffic? Well, it sure doesn't feel good! Conversely, if someone pays us a compliment, or we to them, that's a different energetic experience, isn't it? So I started to pay attention to the spoken word as well as the inner, unspoken dialogue. That required that I pay attention to words, selecting them more carefully.

I've always been so impressed with those individuals and professionals who can craft articulate sentences and clearly convey their thoughts and ideas effortlessly, as if the words are flowing through them, and their mouths and vocal chords are simply an instrument of a greater power. More impressive are those who actually convey and evoke a certain energy with their words. Something interesting came to mind: I suppose the purpose of words is to assign definition, to convey meaning, or describe differences and similarities. But what about translating energy? We select words from our known language that best convey the essence of the feeling, emotion or message we are trying to convey, so words express the energy we either hold or want to convey. Think about a motivational speech, a presidential speech, where words are carefully selected to translate a certain energy.

Now on my new kick about spoken statements, I began to examine further. The reason we don't want to think or speak in the negative is because what we say (just as what we think) is where our attention and energy goes on a subconscious level. So, what about when we ask a question? Then the same must be true. So, if you ask yourself, "Why am I always broke?" your mind will start looking for reasons as to why you lack money. If you ask, "Where is my wallet?" you will begin to try to remember where you left your wallet. So then, what if you ask a positive question? What if we ask, "What would I feel like if I were a tremendous success?" or, "How can I achieve my goals?" or, "What if I was handed an unexpected large sum of money?" I began to tinker with these concepts.

I didn't delve too deep, but just continued to contemplate and conjure up even more things to consider.

The 2016 holiday season proved to be a far livelier than that of 2015! I moved to a new place in early December. I left Buddy with a neighbor for a couple of days so that I could get moved in and have all his things in place. When he arrived, he would feel right at home. I moved on a Saturday and the new washer and dryer were delivered at 10:00 a.m. Monday. The installers assessed the laundry area for a minute and then completed the installation. When finished, they looked around at my place and commented on the decor, especially the Christmas decorations. "Thank you," I said. "I love decorations at the holidays." "How long have you lived here?" inquired one of the men. "Two days," I replied. "Two years?" "No, two days." There was a long silence. They were dumbfounded and amazed. There were no moving boxes anywhere. Things were neat and uncluttered. They could not believe it was possible for any human being to fully move in, with no evidence of a move, in two days! I must say, I was pretty impressed as well. The movers had also mentioned that they've never seen anyone unpack as quickly as I had.

I was fully moved in and the place looked great. Buddy adjusted very well, and quickly staked out what would be "his" areas throughout the house. I was so excited to be in my new space and feeling happy again. I learned a great lesson this Christmas season: Never ever, ever move so quickly and by yourself! Ask for help! My back would pay me in pain currency for months to come. Even so, this was, once again, the most wonderful time of the year!

CHAPTER FOURTEEN

NO PAIN, NO GAIN

*"Meditation trains the mind the way that
physical exercise strengthens the body."*
-Sharon Salzburg

March, 2017. One year since surgery, and I was still in extreme pain in my low back, feet and glutes. I now also had pain in my neck. I had seen two podiatrists, two chiropractors, a sports medicine doctor, a functional medicine doctor, and three orthopedic doctors. I had also been to three physical therapists, one whom specialized in neurological issues. None of them could figure it out. I continued with regular massage sessions, and that provided some relief. Sara was my massage therapist, and we had very similar interests. During massages, we would talk about myofascial release, trigger point therapy, applied kinesiology, quantum physics, and our favorite authors and mentors. She was a bright light and was very methodical, careful to fully understand my situation, and considered what my physical therapist was working on so that her services could be as complementary and synergistic as possible. She was not simply giving me a massage, she was a true healer. Unfortunately, the relief I experienced from her sessions was temporary—a couple of days typically.

I noticed around this time that I had fallen out of my meditation practice again. But I just had too much going on. I didn't have time. I would get to it. I was healing myself in other ways. I told myself that once I addressed the problem with my back, I'd start meditating again. Those were the limiting beliefs I was telling myself, and my self was believing all of them.

Eventually, I scheduled an appointment with a very well-respected spine and neurosurgeon in the Raleigh-Durham area. I was optimistic. I arrived twenty minutes early to complete the requisite paperwork. The staff was pleasant, and escorted me to a room, where a nurse met me. She was also pleasant, genuine. After checking my vitals, she led me to the office of a radiology technologist, who took some images of my back and then escorted me back to the room. A tall bald man in a white coat entered. He said he was sorry for what I was going through. His voice was very soft and soothing. He had wonderful bedside manner. After some discussion, he suggested a myelogram procedure to identify any abnormalities in the spine, spinal cord, or surrounding structures. This is an outpatient test. Dye is injected into the spinal canal through a hollow needle and then images are taken with a CT scan to see if there is a tumor, infection, arthritis, or other abnormalities that are causing pain. I agreed to the procedure and we scheduled it for two weeks later.

The staff at Rex Hospital were just wonderful. I was brought to the first room, where I laid on a table while a doctor injected the dye into my spinal canal. Bizarre electrical pulses pinged in various parts of my legs and feet. It was such an odd feeling. I was trying to separate myself from my body, to be the observer of what was happening—I was getting pretty good at this skill. I was amused by the peculiar sensations I was experiencing and chuckled now and then at the experience. The doctor and his assistant were amused. They'd never witnessed anyone laughing during this procedure. They said they admired my attitude.

After the CT scan was performed, they rolled me into the hallway. I began to feel a little nauseous (common side effect), and overall just off. The feeling of confusion was intensifying. I was rolled around the corner to a recovery room and transported to a bed, where they told me I'd rest for about a half-hour. I continued to feel very weak, but I needed to use the restroom. I was extremely unbalanced and nearly passed out. As I lost my footing, a nurse was passing by and caught me. She got me back to the bed and asked if I wanted to call anyone. I phoned my friend Reilly.

By this time, I literally felt like I was dying and I couldn't speak to him. I couldn't move or talk, and I was desperately trying to keep my eyes open for fear that, if I closed them, I would die. Two nurses rushed over to my bed and started taking vitals. My blood pressure had plummeted. One of the nurses grabbed the phone and said to Reilly, "She can't talk right now," and abruptly hung up my cell phone before throwing it down on the bed. I saw concern on the nurse's face as she gestured something to the other nurse and, in moments, a third nurse arrived. This frightened me, but I was so disoriented, I couldn't respond. I heard someone say they were trying to locate the doctor. After some time (I have no idea how long, I had lost all sense of time), the doctor arrived. He explained that what I was experiencing was a vasovagal episode, which can cause fainting and unconsciousness due to low blood flow to the brain. These episodes are fairly harmless, but they can be a bit frightening.

A couple days later, my spine doctor called to tell me the results of the myelogram. I excitedly answered the phone. *I knew he would find something!* But he didn't. The test results were normal. Completely normal. I was disappointed. He suggested I return in one week to discuss next steps. His nurse would call me in the morning to schedule.

I returned to his office the following Tuesday. By that time, I had severe neck pain again and I let him know. He looked exactly as he did the first meeting: tall, bald and gentle. This time, though, he seemed hasty, in a hurry. He quickly explained that he was certain I needed a second surgery to include another fusion at L5/S1 and a laminectomy. His nurse would contact me later in the day to schedule something in the next two weeks. He exited the room and poked his head back in for a brief moment, "Oh, and about your neck, I don't have a clue." For a moment, I sat confused and confounded by his words. And then, a giant "NO!" immediately exploded into my mind's eye and I ran the heck out of there. Was he even sure surgery was necessary? Aren't there other things we can try? Why so sudden? Did he just want to make a buck off of me? No way would I go through this again. I was done. This was the END. NO MORE!

In that very moment, I realized that I had control and I fully *believed* that my body could heal itself. In that moment, I made some very clear decisions:

1. I was no longer going to be at the mercy of health professionals (who are very well-intentioned), rather I would take my health and state of wellbeing into my own hands.

2. I would immediately radically change my diet to include only organic non-GMO food, supplements, and juicing three to four times a day to reduce inflammation.

3. I would get back into a regular meditation practice, and

4. I would only act in ways that created a positive benefit (no more junk food, no more negative people, a better bed for my back, doing things that brought me joy on an hourly, daily basis, healthier choices all around).

Within four to six weeks of those decisions, my pain level had decreased by about sixty percent! Unfortunately, the level of improvement wasn't sustainable. I decided to try another approach. I began to envision what it felt like to be pain-free. Every day, I sent these messages to my body. On a long weekend, I meditated for three hours Friday, three hours Saturday, and two hours on Sunday, using visualization to display a perfectly happy and healthy lower spine. At one point, late in the afternoon on Monday, I realized that I had been pain-free for two days for the first time in over two years. Once again, an event commanded my attention. I had, on my own, without the help or introduction of medicine, with nothing but my thoughts, or lack of them, rid myself of pain. The simple yet very powerful act of calming my mind changed my reality within a few days. Incredible! If that didn't convince me of the power of meditation, what would?

Meditation relaxes us and takes us into calmer, more relaxed brainwaves. There are five types of brainwaves with varying frequencies:

Higher

* **Gamma** – problem solving, consciousness, perception (40 hz)

* **Beta** – cognition, decision making, active thought, concentration (13-39 hz)

* **Alpha** – calm, relaxed and alert (7-13 hz)

* **Theta** – deep meditation, relaxation, REM sleep (4-7 hz)

Low

* **Delta** – deep dreamless sleep, loss of body awareness (<4 hz)

We tend to exist in a constant state of beta, or high beta, even gamma waves, in active thinking, concentration, and problem solving. So unless we take time to meditate, breathe and relax, we tend to live predominantly in the beta state from the time we awake until the time we go to sleep at night. When we are in a state of stress, anxiety, fear or analysis, we are operating in beta or high beta wave levels.

In this state, we are not open to possibility thinking, to creating, to allowing. Meditation helps to decelerate the beta waves and relax us into alpha, even theta, waves, where our creativity can blossom. In terms of creating your new reality, this is absolutely essential to the transformation, the metamorphosis. Meditation uses the tenants of quantum physics to help us envision possibilities through our subconscious mind. It is the act of allowing ourselves to create new realities through the lack of forced thought—allowing thoughts free of judgment or restriction to build parallel dimensions of possibility in our minds. In this way, a meditation practice can liberate you from perceived expectations, helping you to understand the larger meaning behind whatever it is you are going through.

Access to the subconscious through meditation is also significant in terms of connecting with our limiting beliefs, as five percent of those beliefs reside in the conscious mind and ninety-five percent reside in the subconscious. In order to get to our thoughts in the subconscious, we need to break through our analytical mind and move from beta to alpha and theta waves in the subconscious. Meditation allows us to do this.

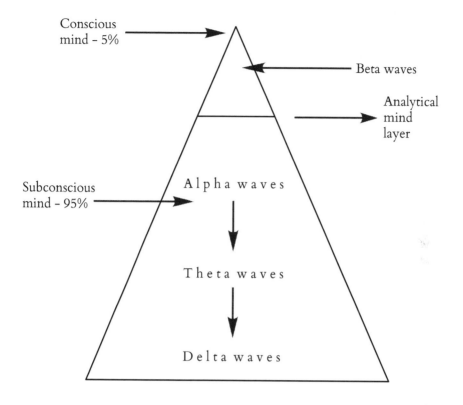

Meditation often involves focusing on something, whether that be an image, an object, sound, or the breath. Transcendental meditation is the most widely known and scientifically studied, but there are numerous forms. Whatever the form, there are a myriad of benefits, including lower blood pressure, decreased anxiety and depression, decreased chronic pain, elimination of toxins, decreased levels of cortisol (stress hormone), increased levels of serotonin and melatonin (calming hormones), improved sleep, better weight control, improved cognition, memory and focus, enhanced work productivity, self-confidence, and less need for medical care and hospitalization. And this is an abbreviated list!

Clearly, slowing down and meditating is good for the mind and mindset. But how exactly does this practice help in guiding you into the new identity you are creating and help you stay there? When we meditate, we are moving beyond our analytical mind and connecting with our consciousness, our pure source energy; we are re-familiarizing ourselves with ourselves.

We also move beyond time when we meditate. In meditation, time does not exist as we know it, and we lose all track of time in the lower frequency states.

I often use meditation as a problem-solving technique. For example, if I feel stuck and unable to find an answer to a particular problem or question, I meditate, even if just for a few minutes, it is helpful, and a nap can work just as well. Taking the analytical mind and brain out of the equation really helps to release any resistance to the issue at hand and allows the answers to flow to us.

EXERCISES:

- Sit or lay down in a comfortable position. If you're wearing them, remove your glasses and watch. Close your eyes gently. Breathe in fully through your nose, and hold for a moment before breathing out through either your nose or mouth. You may also breathe out mostly through your nose and slightly through your mouth. Focus on your breathing. As thoughts come into your mind, just acknowledge them and let them go.

- Do the same as above, but visualize something peaceful, such as a lake on a mountain top, or the sun shining on a calm ocean, or a beautiful, green, unending field. As thoughts come through, again, simply acknowledge and release them.

For each of the exercises above, remain in meditation for at least ten minutes, but optimally for twenty minutes. Notice how you feel, how your body feels. Does your energy feel more balanced? Do you feel calmer, more relaxed? Did you lose track of time? Did you forget about your problems for a bit? Did a solution, answer, or idea come to you during or shortly after meditation? Build up to thirty minutes or an hour at a time.

CHAPTER FIFTEEN

DON'T LOOK BACK
(You're not going that way.)

*"You can't have a better tomorrow if you
are thinking about yesterday all the time."*
-Charles F. Kettering

It was now May, 2017, and my boss at the time requested a one-on-one meeting. It was a highly transitional time for the company. Merger talks were underway. There were a lot of personnel changes. Morale was suffering. A potentially highly stressful period. Very early into our meeting, my boss leaned back in his chair, chewed on his pencil, and said, "Are you looking for another job?"

"No," I answered.

"Hmmm," he said, and paused a few seconds before continuing, "I can't read you."

"Are you trying?" I asked.

"Well," he said, "You just seem so happy and calm and collected."

"Well, I am happy," I responded.

"Even with all the stuff that's going on and what David is up to?"

"Well," I began, "my happiness here is not conditional upon the strategic business decisions the CEO is going to make."

He froze in his chair, put his pencil to his lips, and just said, "Huh." Then he laughed. "Okay then! Wish I could say that!"

I remember thinking to myself, *I did it! I had finally found a way to be happy in an environment that was full of fear-based motivation.* This was no coincidence. I had been telling myself a new story about work, and working on changing my perception of my environment since I couldn't change the environment itself. I was also meditating, exercising appreciation, and remained 100% committed to my own transformation. It just kept getting better and better!

I had become so happy with myself that work took on an entirely different feeling. I can only liken it to when you fall in love and all is right with the world. You still have the same crappy job as you did the day before, but you are high on life, and your body is releasing chemicals like dopamine and oxytocin, and you forget all about your boss, the tedious reporting requirements, that co-worker that annoys you, whatever it may be that previously got under your skin.

By June, I was really starting to feel much better on so many levels. It was a hot summer day, and I had taken a personal day as I had a number of personal items to catch up on. Before going on my walk, I was planning on de-cluttering and identifying as much clothing, books, anything I could donate to Goodwill. I started in the second bedroom. That bedroom houses a fairly large closet and I managed to rid myself of roughly half of the clothes, as well as a number of comforters, a few pillows, bed sheets, and about eight pairs of boots I could no longer wear. I was pulling items from the closet and resting them in strategic piles on my futon. With the last pile in hand, I turned to head over to the futon for the final trip when the adjacent bookcase caught my eye. I gently placed the clothing items down and walked closer to the bookcase, and what I saw gave me a revelation.

Now, throughout my life and corporate career, I have continued to study numerous modalities of healing, a wide variety of approaches to health, and maintained side jobs or hobbies that allowed me to help others and continue my apprenticeship learning (for example, teaching children's yoga and personal training) In the last few years, I donated three bookcases full of books, and then sold the bookcases. Now, I was down to only three bookcases. They were filled with books on Ayurveda, herbal remedies, food and mood, acupuncture, applied kinesiology, meditation, breathing, a few different languages (Spanish, Swahili, Italian—languages have always sparked my interest because they allow you to connect with people whom you otherwise could not). The shelves were also lined with books on quantum physics, consciousness, intention, mind-brain-body connection, plant-based nutrition, Zen Buddhism, Qi-Gong, and so on. Then, in the right corner on the bottom shelf, on one of the bookcases, there were three books dedicated to business. Well, that visual told me A LOT! Up until that time, I only knew that I wanted to be a better version of me. I knew I wanted to help people. I knew I wanted to connect with people. I knew I wanted to be compassionate. To that point, though, I did not know the specifics of what that "new me" looked like, but suddenly I knew and felt, in full sensation, what it looked like in my mind and what it felt like in my body. In that moment, I knew what I had to do.

The golf course community where I had moved to last December is also ideal for walking. It is so serene and has such a pleasant view—undulating greens, lakes, herons, turtles, so soothing and peaceful. There are a lot of dogs in this community, and I love to say hello to any dog who enjoys the interaction. I would often walk with a big smile on my face. I had honestly become that happy! This warm, sunny day, I was doing my usual practices while I walked when the vision of the bookcases entered my mind. I laughed at first, but then I was inspired to make the call that changed everything. I enrolled in a year-long intensive health coach training. I had always wanted to go through this particular program. I love the curriculum. I love the approach. I love the teachers. I really admire the founder and his story. I made the call. I enrolled. I hung up the phone, and a wave of truth washed over me. This felt right in my mind and body, and I suddenly felt such incredible, powerful, and freeing congruence, such alignment. I had no idea where the curriculum would take me, but it was clear that it was the right decision.

One week later, the bank had a sudden mandatory bank-wide call. We were merging and most of us would be out of a job by November 1, 2016. Coincidence, or congruence?

We exist moment to moment, in the split-second present moment, and by the time we are aware of that moment, it has already slipped into the past. In that sense, then, the only thing that really exists at all times is the future. So, we must embrace the idea letting go of our past in order to soar into our new future. If you want a brighter future, you simply need to start living and being that brightness of future possibilities. Now that I had determined the version of me that I wanted to be, there was no turning back. As I was already learning, moving forward into a new future would require *letting go* of my past, my old thoughts, behaviors, and patterns that no longer served me. If I remained focused in the rearview, I would never move forward in any meaningful way. Moving into a new future requires we let go of our past memories, or at least the emotions and beliefs we've attached to those memories, especially memories that trigger negative emotions. When we can do that, well, that is where wisdom is born—when we can have memories without emotional charge.

Creating a new, better, brighter reality then requires letting go of the self you know as you, stepping out of the past, and soaring fully into the future. Of course, we can learn from our past, but we do not exist there.

Letting go also means letting go of fear and worry. I am a recovering perfectionist. I used to worry about everything. I kept to-do lists everywhere. I had to have the "right" job, the nicest clothes, the best soirees, the list goes on. I always had to achieve the highest performance reviews at work and get the highest bonuses. After the economic downturn in 2008, I was part of a team of consultants that went out to regional community banks, helping find appropriate merger partners and/or assisting in a special assets capacity. By the end of 2013, that sector had pretty much dried up and I was out of work. During a conversation with my mom, I said, "I've never been in this position where I had to worry about money before. I hate it." Mom replied, "What do you mean? You've always had a reason to worry, but you've always chosen not to because you had faith it would work out." Wow. She was absolutely correct. In that moment, I knew that a limiting lack belief about money was emerging, and worrying about lacking money would result in me lacking money. At the very least, it certainly would not help me in making or attracting more money. So right there, in that moment, I debunked the belief and let go of the worry. Two weeks later, a former client called and offered me a full-time job. Sometimes we just have to trust that the universe will hear our call, and then get out of our own way and let it answer.

IMPACT IMPERATIVE #5
REPETITION/PRACTICE

I don't care how much you observe, how much you learn, how many elevated emotions you feel, how much appreciation you declare and practice, nothing will change unless you repeat, practice and implement. It is through this repetition that what you learn becomes second nature, automatic, habitual, routine. It is just as the student becomes a concert pianist over time, and becomes one with the instrument as if it has become second nature, or as you have been driving your car for so long that when you step behind the wheel, the process of driving becomes quite automatic. When you combine what you learn with repetition, you create new neural networks and an entirely new level of mind, with neurons firing in new ways. And neurons that fire together, wire together. So, you are replacing the old with the new, and when this starts to happen, you are going to pay attention. You are going to take notice. Your new state of being will make you want to continue to learn, appreciate, repeat, redesign your mind. You will literally begin to lose your old level of mind (Yes, you will lose your mind!), because those old neurons are no longer firing together and wiring together.

CHAPTER SIXTEEN

WHO DO YOU THINK YOU ARE?
(And is that who you want to be?)

*"Your gifted purpose here on earth is to live out
your days bringing and being your best self."*
-Bethanee Epifani

Back in January of 2016, I made the definitive decision that I would make a meaningful change. I did not know the specifics, but I continued to do the practice. Over time, the specifics began to present themselves and I began to allow them to flow to me. Another interesting thing happened: I literally became someone else, or better stated, fully merged with myself.

Now, we are all constantly evolving and are never the same physical being day-to-day. How could we be? Billions of cells in our bodies are continually being replaced each day, while our personalities tend to remain fairly constant over time. But through this process and the belief in the process, my personality actually did change, or at least aspects of it did. When we shed those beliefs that no longer serve us and replace them with more positive and purposeful thoughts and beliefs, we literally alter the chemistry and circuitry in our brain, and we will quite literally become a different person over time. But this new self is not some foreign, unfamiliar self. Quite the contrary! This is actually our authentic self that we have been resisting and keeping away through unexamined, redundant, negative thought. The practice simply allows us to reconnect with and merge fully back into our authentic being.

We all have a great capacity for change within us, but change of any kind can be hard. And sometimes when we decide to make a change, our body and mind can spaz out a little as this new direction is unfamiliar and there is resistance to it. We then tend to say things like, "Yeah, I don't need to change because how I am now feels right," but it's important that we not confuse what feels "right" with what feels familiar.

Have you ever noticed that when you make a decision to do something different and have no resistance to it, no negative belief toward it, it can be an amazing, fun experience? For example, in the spur of the moment, on a beautiful autumn day, you decide to take the back roads to work. The leaves are beautiful and your brain is responding, triggering creativity centers, releasing feel-good hormones and neurotransmitters, and you have a wonderful driving experience. By the time you get to work, you are in such a great state of mind that nothing can bother you. You aren't even a bit concerned that you have arrived a few minutes late—you are ready for the day!

Now, take the same example of taking the back roads, except in this example, there is an accident on the road leading to the highway and you are forced to take the back roads. It's a beautiful autumn day, however, because you were forced to change direction after heading toward the freeway, you have now lost twelve minutes and you don't want to be late. This creates some stress and you don't even notice the beautiful foliage surrounding you as you speed along. You notice that you hit every single red light on your sprint to the office. (You may have hit all the red lights in the first scenario, but were appreciative of them because they allowed you to soak and linger in the scenery a little longer.) You arrive at the office three minutes late and are stressed out. You are incredibly annoyed and it's only 8:12 a.m. What makes the second scenario so different is embedded negative thoughts about being late for work.

I offer this very simple example to illustrate how we may have very different experiences in similar circumstances when we introduce resistance or negative thinking. When we hold no resistance, we are in a completely different state of mind, more of a "go with the flow" mental state, where we open ourselves up to enjoying the journey, as in the first scenario, rather than focusing on the destination. But when we do have resistance, we are too focused on what we need to do and the time and environment in which we need to do it, creating stress, and a far less enjoyable experience, as in the second scenario.

When I decided to start redesigning my mind, I initially worked very hard on transforming my limiting beliefs and meditating on my future version of me. When I started to feel some substantial changes, though, I realized that a meaningful metamorphosis would require more than letting go of thoughts, behaviors and habits that no longer served me—it would also require that I let go of any attachment to what others thought about me. That would be conditional living and would only keep me anchored in the past.

I believe that I also recognized, on some level, that my mindset would not be the only change that would take effect. My personality was changing. My actions and behaviors were changing. The company I kept was changing. I was letting go of the past. All of these changes needed to take place, and there was no way they wouldn't.

I was now letting go of the old behaviors and traits that no longer, and probably never, served me. I was teaching myself to navigate through any anxiety, worry, and fears that impacted my mental health. I fully believed it was possible, and I could feel what that new person looked like, felt like. The specifics were coming more and more into focus as I did the work. That knowing—that belief that a dedication to my mental hygiene was of paramount importance—provided me incredible certainty and assurance about moving forward toward that new version of myself, and I never looked back. On a cellular level, I was morphing out of the former me, the old me, and into the authentic self. I was no longer the Lynn I had told myself I was all those years. And over time, a funny thing happened. I started to follow my bliss, really follow my passion, for the first time ever. The moment I made *that* decision, it felt like pure truth. It was as if I was instantly becoming closer to my true self and essence again.

Now, if you don't want to be the best version of you, that's absolutely okay. This is your journey to experience as you wish. But for those of us who do want to be the best version of ourselves, the self-realized and self-actualized version, ask yourself the following:

1. Do I want to be the best version of me?

2. Do I believe my thoughts impact my feelings and life experience?

3. Do I take a few minutes before going to sleep to deliberately set my intentions for the next day and then wake up deliberately creating my experience through positive and possibility thinking?

(Remember how you felt when you were young on Christmas Eve and Christmas morning, or every day of summer vacation that was filled with hope and great anticipation? Compare that feeling to how you feel when you wake each day.)

Most of us get tripped up on the third question. No doubt that most of us strive to be our best, and most of us really do believe that the way we think directly effects how we feel and experience our lives. But how many of us use deliberate thought to create that better version of ourselves? How can we get up each day and repeat the same set of thoughts, behaviors and attitudes, and expect something to magically change for us? That is the definition of insanity, yes? Remember the movie *Groundhog Day* with Bill Murray? He woke up on the same side of the bed each day, the same song, I Got You Babe, played on the alarm clock that went off at exactly the same time each day. He followed the same route to work each day, passed the same insurance agent, Ned Ryerson, and on it went. Don't we do the same thing? We get out of our bed the same way, follow our normal breakfast routine, check social media, the news, go the same way to work, sit in the same chair, see the same people, go home, eat, go to sleep, repeat. When we awake each morning, we immediately begin to think about our problems, our deadlines, something our ex did yesterday to annoy us, what we need to accomplish and the time constraints in which that must happen.

So, why do we get so tripped up on this question of using deliberate thought to create our reality? Very likely, because we don't believe it is possible. Maybe we have trouble reconnecting with our true authentic self, or because we live life conditionally, expecting that something needs to happen in order for life to be better, for us to be happier ("Once I have the money," or, "Once I have the relationship"). It's inside out, though, literally. You'll only see it when you believe it. You must believe in something in order to see it manifest, not the other way around.

Or finally, perhaps it is because we have no idea what we would want to create or experience, and, therefore, cannot envision what that self or life even looks or feels like. Relax! You don't have to see all of it in great detail, but you absolutely must be able to feel it. You must have intention behind the vision. People can have positive thoughts all day long, but without belief and intention, nothing will change. For example, you might repeat your affirmation of "I am wealthy" every day, but if you are holding a lack belief about money then you probably don't fully believe in your wealth potential.

I believe that one of the big reasons we get tripped up on this idea of our ability to create our reality is that we don't see ourselves as the creators we are, so we've never even given it any thought. But we ARE creators! First and foremost, each one of us is a creator! Remember when we were young and lived in our imagination almost daily? We created adventures, stories, things, places, and people in our minds and our imagination knew no limitations. Our limitations and restrictions in life are learned over time and self-imposed. We "create" our limitations through our own faulty thoughts and beliefs. They become a kind of contract with ourselves that we've agreed to, but unfortunately, they keep us from being the creators we are. How did the world evolve as it has with industrial, technological, artistic and other improvements? Through creation and co-creation! And that was done by whom? Beings, just like each of us. Creation is in all of us. Isn't that why we're here? To be the best creation we can be? To be (create) the best version of ourselves?

So, who are you and what is the best version of you that you can imagine? What does it look like for you to be living your gift? You may know that you want a career change to best use your God-given gifts or unique talents, and you may know exactly what that change is and feels like, but you have some fear about failure or change itself that is keeping you stuck where you are, otherwise, you'd already have made the change.

If you can't envision the specifics, then simply start with the general feeling or emotion. Do you want to be a more empathetic, compassionate person? How does that feel? Do you wish to have peace? What does that feel like? Do you want to be less angry or less anxious? Whatever those qualities are, feel them as best you can, and don't focus on the material conditions. Remember, it comes from within. Years ago, a colleague asked me, "If you could have one thing in the world, what would it be?"

I answered that I need two things, "I would need a villa off the Amalfi coast, and inner peace. But I need the villa first."

"Why?" he asked.

I answered, raising my eyebrows, as if the answer was obvious, "Well, if I had the inner peace, I wouldn't give a crap about the villa!"

Many of us, when thinking about what would make us a happier, better version of ourselves, say something like, "I'd be happier if I had more money," or, "When I find the right partner, I'll be happier," but this is conditional living—waiting for or depending on an external, often material thing, event, person, opportunity or circumstance to play out as you wish so that you can feel happy or blissful or fulfilled. That's placing the onus on everyone and everything to bring pleasure to you, rather than finding your own bliss within, and then allowing those things, events, people, opportunities or circumstances to flow to you.

CHAPTER SEVENTEEN

A NEW BEGINNING (or era)

"New beginnings are often disguised
as painful endings."
-Lao Tzu

The health coach curriculum began in July, 2017. By now, I was walking five to six miles a day. I was in a constant state of bliss. I used that time to listen to the lectures. Between lectures, I continued with my other exercises, like "Walking into My Future," "Appreciation Alphabet Soup," and others. I found the modules to be fairly easy, yet thrilling at the same time. I had been studying for fun my entire life and was passionate about health and wellness. When I wasn't listing to the lectures, I was listening to other industry leaders in biology, belief, conscious leadership, positive mindset, epigenetics, quantum physics, energy balancing, and healing. I was also incredibly fascinated by how this process of my own mind redesign had impacted me. With that in mind, I began soaking up as much knowledge as I could on the topic. I was a sponge for lectures about toxic thinking and the effects on our health and our life experience. I was in my zone, my vortex. Every day provided an amazing experience. I had no expectation of where this all was taking me or what the outcome would be, but I was thoroughly enjoying the process. It was FUN!

I continued to listen to Dr. Joe Dispenza's lectures, and sought out a number of other teachers as well that spoke about transformation and the power of shifting thoughts, beliefs and behaviors. For whatever reason, this was becoming increasingly resonant and important to me. I didn't question it. It was exciting to me, and that was enough for me. I knew that if I followed my passion, good things would happen—still like a dog with its head out the window! I immediately began attempting to redesign my mind and my self even further.

I was excelling in the curriculum and the modules came quite easily to me. This did not feel like studying at all. It was pure enjoyment. I had studied the subject matter my entire life, but now, *wait a minute, I'm finally following my passion!* This was a new beginning for me, although I had no idea or expectation of what the outcome of the curriculum would be. I just knew I needed to follow down this path. I aced the first test in October, and was making a lot of friends, meeting like-minded people, and just creating a really great supportive network of colleagues. It was a bit of a balancing act given that I was still working at the bank and could only study at night and during the lunch hour. And it was a stressful time at the bank—continued and heightened discussions about a potential merger had some people in a bit of a panic. We had all been notified about the merger in June, but now the official transaction was imminent.

The merger was officially announced on November 1, 2017. My boss had let me know in September that my position would not be eliminated in November as originally anticipated, so I had a bit of cushion. By this time, morale at the bank was through the floor. People highly distrusted those at the top, and there was a lot of bad mouthing going on, at all levels. I was fortunate that I was now working remotely most of the time, so I could just focus on my work and not need to deal with any negative morale.

Right around this time, I had a meeting with a local attorney to discuss a workout that involved a bankruptcy. Midway through the conversation, and without any logical segue at all, the attorney put his pen down, leaned back into his office chair, and declared, "Lynn. My God. How on earth did you get through all you've had to endure? How did you do it, just you, by yourself? It's really quite remarkable. I don't know how you got through it so well." I felt tears begin to well up in my eyes and a voice was trying to amplify enough for the tears to hear, *Stay professional! Don't cry!* I replied simply, "I think I must have had some help from the universe, God, angels, others, or all of the above, because I honestly don't know." He said, "Well, I'm impressed. I'd probably be one big stress case. I don't know how you've been holding up so well."

But in spite of everything, juggling the curriculum with work, merger and associated tensions, and still trying to rid myself of some ongoing back pain, I did not feel stressed, until... an event in December, 2017. A deadline that was coming due made me realize that I was holding a pretty strong limiting belief about something. I had a new boss, and I really wanted to make a good impression. This deadline had just been announced. I was having a very somatic response—my body was very tense, I felt irritable, I was jittery, nauseous. It was literally making myself sick. Mostly, I had a tremendous amount of fear about this assignment. My body was definitely providing me information through the feelings I was experiencing. And the strength of my body's response told me that the underlying limiting belief had already gained a lot of momentum. Chances were, given my body's response, I had been resting my attention on a negative thought or belief for some time. So, I immediately checked in. I stepped away from my work and asked myself, "What on earth are you so stressed out about?" My answer was the deadline. I did this little exercise I call "So What?" I had identified that the deadline was causing me stress, but I had to go a little deeper. What about the deadline was making me uncomfortable? I recognized that it was fear-based, but what about this deadline produced fear in me? I was afraid I might miss it. I began the following coaching session with myself:

Okay, SO WHAT if I miss the deadline? Answer: They (the new company, in particular, my boss) might not like me. Okay, SO WHAT if they don't like you? Answer: They might fire me. Okay, SO WHAT if they fire you? Answer: I will be out of work. Okay, SO WHAT if you are out of work? Answer: I may not be able to pay the bills. Okay, SO WHAT if you can't pay the bills? Answer: I could lose my home.

And when I got to that point, I did two things. First, I laughed at the hilarity of it all. I had created this fear in my own mind. Next, I reality tested. Going to the beginning and end of the exercise I asked myself if have I ever missed a deadline. No, was the answer. Have I ever been unable to pay the bills, or lost my home? No. So, clearly, I was holding on to a fear-based limiting belief that I created myself, and that was not at all based in reality. Once I completed this simple exercise, my mind and body were completely relaxed, my anxiety and tension were fully released. I was free (and yes, I met the deadline).

Shifting the limiting belief could not have happened when I first felt the somatic stress response, as there was too much momentum from the negative thought. The process of peeling the layers back actually helps to slowly reduce and ultimately eliminate the resistance, the momentum generated by the lack or limiting belief, and that is when change can occur.

Many organizations breed a culture of fear-based motivation rather than inspired action. We've all been trained at an early age to get good grades, do well on tests, to please our teachers, parents, others. Many of us choose college courses and concentrations that will please our parents, not ourselves. And career choices are often based on what others feel we should do with our lives, not what passion we wish to follow. Our lives become conditional upon what others think of us. Those of us who follow our passion and choose that perfect career for ourselves find that it creates an inspired state of mind. Unfortunately, many of us, many of you who are reading this book, continue simply going through the motions, year after year, feeling uninspired and empty. And yeah, it can be really difficult to make a change, but change is possible. But let's assume for a moment that change is not possible. Then what? Well, if you can't change your career environment, you can certainly and very effectively change your perception of and reaction to your career environment, just as I had.

And consider this simple question: What were you thinking?! What were you thinking when you woke up yesterday? ("Oh crap. Deadline. I don't want to get up.") What were you thinking when you woke up this morning? ("Oh no, don't want to go to work!") How many minutes, or seconds, passed between the time you hit the alarm and the time you grabbed your phone to check texts, Twitter, Instagram, Facebook? ("Oh, Sherri's doing yoga again. She's so thin and pretty and I'm gross." "Trish and Tom on vacation again? My life sucks." "I can't believe no one liked my post! It was funny.... well, maybe I'm not so funny... no one likes me.") And what were you thinking when you turned on the TV and saw another breaking alert about a mass shooting or natural disaster or that the stock market plummeted, or that the government is in crisis? ("Oh, we are so screwed!") What were you thinking when you got in traffic? ("My ex-wife or husband is so annoying!" "STOP TEXTING AND DRIVING!") And by the time you get to work, you're in a crappy mood, you go to the same desk, drink the same weak coffee, see the same co-workers, and by association, you think to yourself, "My job stinks." But is it really your job that stinks? Or is it your thoughts?

So, the question is: are we really that dissatisfied with our jobs and careers, or just the meaning we've attached to them?

EXERCISES:

- Try the "So What" exercise. Is there something causing you anxiety? Is there an underlying fear? Try peeling the layers back to get to the root of the limiting belief. Next, reality test. Were you able to disarm the momentum and power of the belief?

- For the next seven days, pay close attention to your thoughts as soon as you can upon waking. PAUSE before you start checking social media. If you check it anyway, pay close attention to how your mind and body feel. Is there a subtle increase in tension or anxiety as you compare and despair with others on social media, or as you feel you need to delete the numerous emails that came through while you slept? Whatever it is, pay attention to how you feel in body and mind.

CHAPTER EIGHTEEN

NET OPERATING ENERGY (energy balance)

*"Balance is the key to everything. What we do,
think, say, eat, feel, they all require awareness,
and through this awareness, we can grow."*
-Koi Fresco

Happy or not in our career, work can be stressful. Let's face it. It's often difficult to find and feel that balance. I know many of us can relate to the stresses that face us in our corporate lives, but we don't *need* to have a stress response to situations *we define* as stressful! At the very least, we don't have to have a prolonged stress response. In my previous example about a deadline that produced anxiety, the somatic response indicated that I had a strong belief about the deadline and, therefore, I attached a definition of "fearful." It was only defined as fearful because of a second belief I had about my abilities (or possible lack of). Things, events, words, circumstances, are inherently neutral, but when we assign them negative meanings, they become problematic. As I'm writing this chapter, my dog has become very ill. If a friend or neighbor's dog were to become ill, I'd likely have a neutral reaction, or a fairly low-level emotional response. But because it's MY dog, my emotional response is significant and prolonged. If you lose a dollar, you don't react with a lot of stress, but if you lost $1,000, you'd likely respond with a stressful reaction, due to a lack belief about money.

Work cultures often have their own definition of stress as being a rite of annual review passage. These cultures are still too common, unfortunately, and they tend to create a collective mindset where the worker bees wear stress like a badge of honor, as if the more stress we can endure, the greater the superhero we are. I used to work for a large accounting firm when I lived in California. A forty-hour work week was unheard of, and truly shameful. No one would ever think of admitting to working only forty hours! I think the minimum work week was probably right around sixty hours, but quite often, many of us worked eighty to a hundred hours or more a week. It was highly encouraged: if we worked eleven hours or more in a given day, we'd get a free dinner of our choice and a town car home. As a junior analyst or manager, that can be quite appealing, intoxicating. I remember a female manager who had just given birth to her third child was working from her hospital bed in the hours just after delivery. Where is the balance?

Maintaining a positive energy balance is really important in maintaining and improving our mindset and overall health. This can be difficult for so many of us, especially given the everyday stress in our work lives, which is where most of our time is spent. Our energy gets compromised every day for many reasons, but we have control over this, too. Our energy is not unlimited. It can increase and decrease, and our available energy on a given day is finite, but there are always ways to improve and increase its bounty. Again, we just need to raise our awareness to our thoughts, actions, and behaviors. As a rule, where we place our attention is where we put our energy. Certain uses of energy can actually enhance our energy balance, while other uses of energy can detract from our energetic reserves. If we are focused on negative people, events, circumstances, or behaviors, our energy will be consumed by the negative, and we'll soon deplete our energy supply.

How do you use your energy? How is your energy level on a given day? What actions enhance or add to your energy in a positive way? What actions do you take that deplete or decrease your energy? Are there patterns? Are there areas for improvement?

Combining my corporate and coaching sides, I began to explain energy balance in terms of an income statement, with income, expenses and NOI, or net operating income, where "energy" replaces "income." If you are operating a business, or if you are evaluating a business as an investment or considering lending based on NOI, you'd want that bottom line NOI to be positive, wouldn't you?

Now think about YOUR NOI, but in terms of energy. Our energy stores, or dollars, if you will, are in ATP units. ATP (short for adenosine triphosphate) is typically referred to as the "molecular unit of currency" that provides us the fuel or energy we need on a daily basis. Now, it is estimated that we twenty-five percent of our energy is expended on powering our brain every day. To put that into perspective, that would be similar to the energy it takes to run a marathon! As part of their training, though, marathon runners always incorporate proper strength training and rest for their muscles, and allow for their energy stores to be replenished. Professional athletes understand that muscles need rest and energy needs restoration.

Our brain is not a muscle, but is often referred to as one. Like other muscles, it will grow and improve the more we use it. Like other muscles, it needs rest and restoration, and like other muscles, it will reach a point of diminishing return when overused. As Alan Cohen said, "There is a virtue in work and there is a virtue in rest. Use both and overlook neither." So, it really is all about balance.

Now going back to our income, or energy, statement, we have energetic income or intake, and energetic expense or expenditure. What are some of the factors that influence our energy balance? Of course, our thoughts, feelings and emotions can influence us in a positive or negative manner. Our lifestyle can be a big factor. This includes our eating habits, the quality and quantity of our diet, our physical activity levels, the amount and intensity (or lack) of physical activity, and our downtime—how much sleep and rest we allow our body and brain on a consistent basis. All of these can add or detract from our energy balance. Other factors include our behaviors, our body weight, hormones, overall health, the environment, and our perception of and reaction to it.

So, let's begin with the income sources. All the things that generate positive energetic revenue streams to you are your energy income sources. All the ways you use or expend your energy negatively are your expenses. You want your NOE (net operating energy) to always be positive at the end of the day. So think of things or thoughts or actions that impact you positively throughout the day: seeing your spouse, talking with your children, or your parents, meditating for twenty minutes, thinking how appreciative you are for your life, enjoying the drive to your workplace, eating a healthy meal, achieving your goals, whatever it may be. Then assign them a number between one and ten, with ten being the most fulfilling or good use/source of energy. These are things that nourish you in some way, whether it be the food you ingest or other things that provide your mind, body, and spirit nourishment.

Now, do the same for your expenses—things, thoughts, or actions that impact you negatively throughout the day. For example, cursing the driver who cut you off, thinking about how annoyed your ex or co-worker made you the other day, skipping breakfast and lunch because there just wasn't enough time, going through your day in a place of fear or anxiety rather than a place of inspiration, realizing you didn't get any "likes" on your Facebook post. Then assign a negative number from negative one to negative ten, with negative ten being the poorest use of your energy. These are the biggest drains on your energy; these items deplete nourishment to your mind, body, and spirit. Sum the totals, and the sum of income and expenses is your NOE.

Income

Hugs to spouse and children	10
Healthy breakfast	10
Creative collaboration with co-workers	8
Being commended on a project	8
Appreciating my boss and co-workers	7
Good walk with the dog	10
Total Income	53

Expenses

Stressed myself out at work all day	−10
Swore at driver who cut me off	−8
Negative social media	−8
Negative news stories	−10
Pizza and chips for lunch	−10
Stress over newly announced deadline	−10
Overdid my workout	−8
Total Expenses	−64

Net operating energy	−11

As stated, we want our net energetic income to always be positive. So, clearly, this example is not a good bottom line, and this energy statement has a lot of room for improvement. Now, how did this person get to the numbers they assigned to the entries? Would you have assigned different ratings on your own NOE statement? Most definitely. This is because we all have unique individual beliefs about the items we list, how we may react to certain situations based on these beliefs, and the amount of momentum we allow to follow each action or circumstance. For example, let's take that deadline that caused stress in our example above. Here, it is assigned a -10 for pizza and chips. You, though, might actually assign this a -2. Maybe you don't think pizza and chips are so bad because you rarely eat that way, or maybe that meal doesn't make you sleepy an hour later, but for someone else, that same pizza and chips might not be a healthy choice that makes them feel sluggish after eating it, or it may be a choice that makes someone judge themselves, adding negative momentum and negative thought about this one action. Try this exercise on your own and see what your statement looks like. Feel free to make it as simple or complex as you like. You may be surprised at the outcome.

Let's talk a little more about energy, because whatever it is that you focus on, you give your attention to, and is exactly where you expend your energy. As has been discussed, we spend most of our mental energy in negative thinking as soon as we awake each day, focusing on all of our problems and anticipating the future based on our past patterns and behaviors. This pattern of thinking really diminishes our potential creative energy by focusing on the past. Our minds become so crowded with unproductive, energy sapping thoughts, fears, worries, and concerns that there is no room to create our amazing future in our minds. But by shifting this pattern to eliminate the un-serving thoughts, letting go of our worries, fears, and anxious thoughts, we free up space for potential creative energy, allowing us to think of and create a future based on possibilities. We can achieve this by practicing the exercises I've outlined, but also through quieting the mind on a regular basis, through breathing, meditation, and consistent practice of all of these. In the first illustration below, there is clearly no room to create a future because the person is so very stuck in the past, in fear, lack, and in thought patterns that don't serve them.

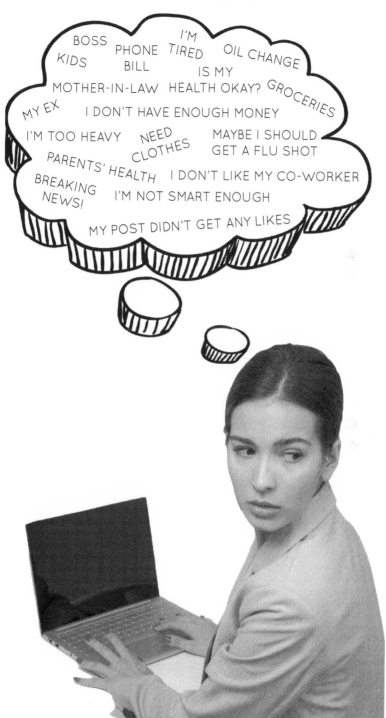

Removing and replacing negative thought patterns with positive thoughts allows room for creative energy and possibility thinking. Of course, we can't always replace 100%!

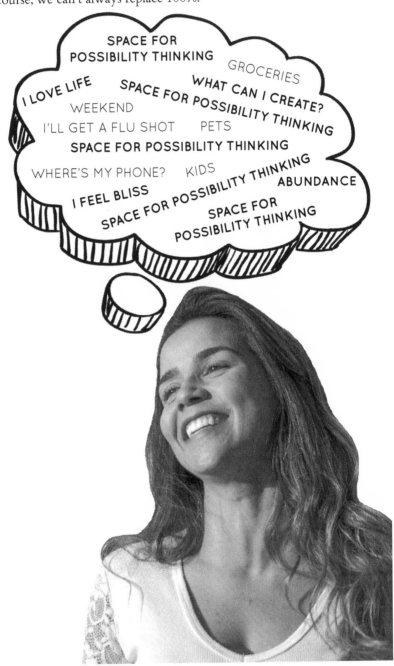

Consider your own thought patterns. Are you constantly thinking of your problems? Do your thoughts impact how you feel? Of course they do. *How* are your thoughts impacting how you feel? Can you free up additional creative potential by eliminating thought patterns that don't serve you? What types of thoughts or activities are impacting your net operating energy's bottom line? What changes can you make immediately that would have a positive impact on your NOE bottom line and your creative energy potential?

EXERCISE:

- Create your own NOE statement. Repeat this exercise a few times a week. Do you notice any patterns? What does your NOE statement reflect?

CHAPTER NINETEEN

THE VOICES IN YOUR HEAD
(Can you hear them?)

"Art is the act of doing work that matters while dancing with the voice in your head that screams for you to stop."
-Seth Godin

As I continued to practice, I began to realize how few of us actually pay attention to our thinking. We are truly physically focused beings. We get sick, we see a doctor. We get a cavity, we go to the dentist. We get a cut, we heal with a disinfectant and Band-Aid. We go to the hairdresser. We wear nice clothes. We go to the gym so we can be strong. We get dirty, we take a shower. We (hopefully) try to eat well. We give so much thought and attention to our physical form, our physical wellbeing, physical comfort, physical appearance, physical performance, physical health, but very rarely do we think about what we are thinking about. If, in the very instant a negative thought popped into our mind, it also emerged as a label in physical form and attached itself to our body or clothing, we'd tear it off in an instant, as the physically oriented beings we are. We surely would not want to be physically cloaked in these negative signs for the world to see now, would we? Yet we are absolutely cloaked (mentally) in these thoughts that directly shape our mindset.

Our mindset consists of a set of attitudes and beliefs that dictate our behaviors or responses to events or situations, and it impacts *everything*: our relationships, our careers, lifestyles, self-care, home environments, everything, and none of them can improve if there exists resistance—some limiting belief about the particular aspect in our mindset. And our daily behaviors can most always be tied back to a belief. If you want to be healthier but refuse to change your diet or quit smoking, there's likely a belief in your hard drive that is creating resistance. Otherwise, you'd have already made the change. What is the belief? (You're not worth it? It's too hard?) If someone blows right through a stop sign and cuts you off driving and you go immediately to rage, there's likely an underlying belief. What is it? (I had to follow the rules growing up and I still do today, so everyone should have to!)

We have beliefs about everything! As a health coach, I often coach people on mindset and beliefs, as this can dictate their level of success in the areas of life they wish to improve upon. For example, give some consideration to what areas are impacted by your negative thoughts, those voices in your head. Is the finance area voice saying, "I'm broke?" Is the career area voice saying, "I hate my job?" Is the education area voice saying, "I'm not smart enough?" Is the physical activity voice saying, "I'm too fat," or, "I don't have time to work out?" What are those voices saying? You can probably identify with a number of voices in various aspects of your life.

Our thoughts directly impact how we feel, and how we feel directly impacts how we think. So, if we want to feel our best then we really need to pay attention to and think about what we are thinking about! Maybe the biggest reason we should pay attention to our thinking is—and this is huge—our thoughts can actually make us sick! We often hear about the power of positive thinking, but what about the power of negative thinking? Negative thoughts are just as powerful, and due to the repetitious and often prolonged stress response, they are far more threatening. Every time we have a thought, there is a chemical, biological response to that thought. For example, when we have a positive thought, our brain releases chemicals, such as dopamine, oxytocin, and other neurotransmitters that send signals to the body, allowing the body to experience a positive feeling. The body then sends a signal back to the brain indicating this good feeling state. But when we have a negative thought, there is a very different chemical reaction in the brain. And when we are having 70,000 to 80,000 thoughts in a given day, as suggested by neuroscience, and most of them negative thoughts, there is an even more redundant feedback loop and prolonged stress response. It's estimated that sixty to seventy percent of us live in a chronic state of elevated stress. That's a frightening statistic, but it isn't difficult to believe or understand, especially in the "high alert" and "breaking news" culture that has developed in recent history.

So, we know where these voices in our head come from and how prevalent they are, so why don't we notice them? As I mentioned, the problem is that roughly ninety-five percent of these beliefs originated and are stored in our subconscious.

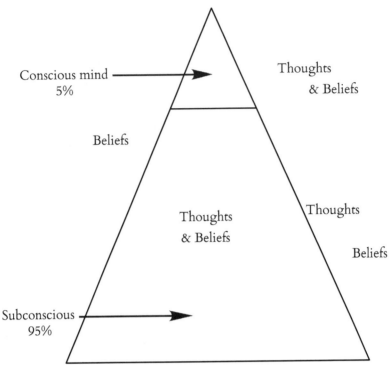

In the isosceles triangle above, the bottom portion is our subconscious. The top portion is our conscious mind. The vast majority of our thoughts and beliefs are stored in our subconscious mind. So, if we are mostly unaware of these thoughts and beliefs then the key to transformation really must be in bringing them into our awareness, or our conscious mind.

We hold beliefs about everything! Our work, our world, even our words. I recently told a coaching client that this transformation takes perseverance, to which she responded, "Ugh." I said, "Wow. Wait a minute. Let's take a look at this because you have a belief system about a word." Now, a word is inherently neutral, as are most things in life before we attach definitions, emotions, and meanings to them.

So I said, "Perseverance is just a word, but you've attached some sort of meaning to it, so let's take a look at that. What does it mean to you?"

She responded, "Well, it's hard, and a lot of work."

That was pretty heavy, so I offered her this, "Well, let's take a look at this. What is perseverance? It's a knowing, a firm belief in something we know is right, true, correct. So, we persevere because our knowledge of something to be right is so unwavering that we simply trust in it, and are willing to simply just keep figuring out a different way to achieve whatever it is we want to achieve, because of that trust, right?" You can see how much lighter that is. It's true that the definition of the word "perseverance" includes "maintained activity or tenacity, despite difficulties, failures or opposition," but we don't have to view obstacles as failures or difficulties, only hurdles and information. We usually persevere because we *believe* in the outcome.

As part of my health coach curriculum, I was practicing coaching a girl who had identified a limiting belief as being afraid that people would witness her failing. Now, there are a couple of different limiting beliefs in there, but I asked her to state that out loud. This session was over the phone, but through the phone lines, I could hear her body contracting and her vocal cords straining. It was hard for her to get the words out of her mouth. And that is exactly what a limiting belief is, right? A belief (a thought repeated over time) that constrains us from being all we can be. So, I asked her, "How did it feel saying that?"

She said, "It felt awful."

"Why? Why is that?" I asked.

And she answered, "Because it's not true."

"Exactly," I said. "It is not true. It is not who you are. It is not who you came here to be." Now that we identified that this belief is untrue, it was time to shift and tell another story. We began to change this story by stating why she is not a failure, and then why she is a success, taking the negative word "failure" out of the discussion entirely. This was a really simple exercise, but a very powerful realization for her. It was also powerful for me, because it validated that I can actually help others with their own poor thinking and limiting beliefs. This brings up an interesting and important note.

Now, these women were not transformed after one session of shifting limiting beliefs, but in each case, there was a profound awareness that allowed for an immediate shift. Our brain has the amazing ability to reorganize the synaptic wiring in response to learning, experience or injury ("neuroplasticity"). We have all been creating our own unique circuitry in response to our individual experiences throughout our life. Our repeated thoughts and behaviors have created our current state of being. Similarly, we can rewire this circuitry and thereby modify our state of being for a more productive, fulfilling experience.

EXERCISES:

- The next time you identify a negative thought, imagine that it is written on your clothing, or there is a bubble above your head that everyone can see. How do you react?

- Try stating the limiting belief out loud. How does it make you feel? Does it lose its power?

- Next time you react to an event, situation or circumstance (or word) in a negative manner, check in. Was the negative reaction truly warranted? (Note: your reaction may be valid, but may not truly be warranted.)

CHAPTER TWENTY

CLEAN UP YOUR CLAN!

*"You cannot expect to live a positive life
if you hang with negative people."*
-Joel Osteen

Just as work can drain our energy, so can people, and they can drain us of more than energy! People can also drain us of time. Have you ever heard the saying that you are the average of the five or so people that you spend the most time with? Have you ever given any consideration to the company you keep and how they impact your mental wellbeing? Who are the five people with whom you spend most of your time? What does the average of that group look like?

I realized fairly early on in my injury that this process, and my healing, would necessitate that I remove any negative people from my energy field, and it was quite possible that my mix of friends and acquaintances would change as a result. I needed to let go of people who were toxic or draining my energy. This didn't bother me. I knew what I had to do. And that knowing gave me the conviction I needed to move forward with my transformation without a care about what anyone thought or expected of me. And interestingly, the better I felt, the more I realized that I simply did not want to be around negative people and their negative thoughts, behaviors, attitudes, and actions. It was far easier than I thought, and just happened naturally, organically. I can liken it to when you change your diet: you start incorporating more nutritious foods into your lifestyle, and one day realize you have changed your body chemistry as a result, and consequently, you no longer have an appetite for unhealthy foods Likewise, as my mind went through its redesign, I didn't have an appetite for negativity, and negativity didn't really have an impact on me any longer. Just like after changing your diet, you can be around sweets and don't feel the need to engage; it will be far easier to be around negative energy because that energy will just ping off of you.

When you start to do the work, you'll automatically begin to experience a shift in yourself—a shift into a truly joyous and blissful state, because you will no longer live conditionally. You will no longer give a rip about what others think about you, and you will no longer have the same tolerance for negativity and victim mentality as you once did. But you will understand and appreciate why they remain in this state, without judgment.

Cleaning up your clan doesn't just refer to people with whom we physically interact. We must also consider our relationship with people and groups on social media. Social media outlets like Facebook and Twitter purport through marketing that these platforms help to bring us together, help us connect with more and more people. And don't get me wrong. Social media has its uses and benefits. For example, if you live in the United States and you have family in Europe, this is a great way to keep in contact, but, in general, as we become more "connected" through social media with the rest of the world, we actually become far more disconnected from ourselves and others.

So when does social media transition from a way to keep in touch to a way to disconnect? Probably when you realize that you are judging someone's cute pictures of their baby's first birthday party. Or when you are comparing and despairing because your life doesn't look even half as interesting as that of your old friend from high school, and you start to ask yourself how your life ended up being so uninspired and boring (Hey! Get out of the past when this happens!), or maybe when you are feeling jealous at someone's vacation pictures. And social media only provides one little snapshot, and we often base our perceptions on this brief imagery.

When we allow social media to influence our behaviors and opinions of ourselves for the worse, we really need to evaluate our relationship with social media, and our beliefs about its value or contribution to our life experience. When you are examining the health of your relationships and how they impact your energy balance and state of mind, don't forget to evaluate your relationship with social media.

Sometimes, these relationships go beyond simply draining our energy; they can be downright toxic and harmful. Further, sometimes we don't even recognize that we are in a toxic relationship until damage has been done. Some tips for navigating negative or toxic relationships:

1. Evaluate the relationship.

Is the relationship draining you of time, energy, or money? Is it creating drama or trauma? Do you feel your esteem suffers or it triggers damaging limiting beliefs within you? Notice how you feel mentally and physically when you are around the person or people in question.

2. Take care of you.

You are the #1 priority, so always put you first. In order to be the very best version of you, you will need to take care of yourself and your energy. Treat your energy as gold and don't let others steal it. Decide if you need to disengage or completely cut someone off; either answer is fine, as long as it is best for you. Practice being the Michelin Man or other tools.

3. Explore means for communicating.

You could record a voice message that says, "Hey, thanks for calling. I'm going through some changes and eliminating negative people from my life now, so if I don't return the call, you may be one of them." But there are probably better alternatives, such as nonviolent communication or conscious communication. Nonviolent communication (NVC) is an approach that utilizes compassion and empathy in communicating unmet needs, rather than defensiveness or aggression. NVC was developed by Marshall Rosenberg in the 1960s. Conscious communication, developed by Deepak Chopra, expands on Rosenberg's work. The key principal in these approaches is simply identifying any need(s) that is/are not being met by the other person, and then communicating that need. The goal is to make it as easy as possible to shift behaviors and better meet each other's needs.

4. Seek out positive relationships.

Certainly, improving our mental hygiene and cleaning up our thinking will go a long way toward increasing our space for creative possibility thinking. In the same way, cleaning up our clan, removing negative people, and aligning with positive people will have the same impact.

EXERCISE:

- Take notice and really assess the people with whom you sur-round yourself on a daily basis, and how they affect your ener-gy during those interactions. Are they mostly positive people? If they tend to be more negative, do you find yourself going to their level, taking on their energy when you are with them? Acting as they would want you to act rather than how you wish to behave? Saying things you normally wouldn't? Do they take you away from your feeling of bliss? If so, you really need to consider changing the mix of people with whom you surround yourself.

IMPACT IMPERATIVE #6
COMMITMENT/DISCIPLINE

As I've stated numerous times before, this takes some effort, some commitment and discipline. Discipline is not a bad word! It is not a prison sentence! But isn't it interesting that so many of us assign a negative meaning to this word (a limiting belief)? It's really just about being consistently committed. All of the greatest athletes, musicians, and CEOs had discipline. Some tips for succeeding in your discipline: don't make excuses, don't listen to those voices in your head, DO acknowledge and celebrate your successes, remain open to the process, stay focused, be patient, be consistent, and believe. If you have trouble with discipline, try starting with baby steps, and remember, this is actually a fascinating and fun creative process! So please enjoy the process!

CHAPTER TWENTY-ONE

BELIEVE IN THE BUTTERFLY

"What the caterpillar calls the end,
the rest of the world calls a butterfly."
-Lao Tzu

B ruce Lipton, Ph.D. provides an amazing description of the transformation of a caterpillar into a butterfly. The caterpillar has seven billion cells. Lipton compares the cells to citizens in an economy, with different groups of cells performing a variety of job functions. The cells in the digestive system are breaking down incoming food and making products out of it, cells in the respiratory system are ensuring that fresh oxygen is being deployed correctly, and there are structures for conveying nutrients throughout the organism, just like highways and transportation systems. Each and every one of the cells has a job to do, and is working hard, and the caterpillar is growing. There is a growing and booming economy within the caterpillar, with working cells at full employment.

There comes a time when the caterpillar reaches maximum capacity and can no longer grow. The caterpillar stops eating, and the cells are now confused. With the reduced eating, there is far less food getting to the cells of the digestive system. There is less and less work for the cells to do, until there is no work at all, as if the cells have been handed pink slips—there is no need for them any longer. Soon, there is less need for jobs in the respiration department, the immune department, and so on, and chaos in the population follows. The cells begin to give up and die off.

But there is a group of genetically identical cells called imaginal cells that are not at all effected by the failing economy. Despite the chaos within the dying caterpillar, these cells have a vision—a vision of a new and sustainable way of life that looks and feels completely different. These cells are committed to the vision. They reorganize around the new vision, and with inspired action, create the new and better version of the being formerly known as the caterpillar. The imaginal cells believe in the butterfly and move from the caterpillar's no longer sustainable way of life into this beautiful new version of life called the butterfly.

Now, Lipton discusses this in the context of the global awakening, comparing the imaginal cells to our collective evolution, moving from a no longer sustainable way of existing into a new and highly sustainable existence. But I think it is really relevant here in this context because of the belief in the vision of the imaginal cells. These cells are 100% committed to the butterfly. They share an absolute knowing in the possibility, the future form, and they trust in it as they work together to co-create the new version. When we make that decision to become the next and best version of ourselves, we need to be able to imagine it, feel it, and fully believe in the possibility. We need to have the same knowing that the imaginal cells in the butterfly have. Now, many of us view possibilities as being outside of who we (think we) are, outside of the character, identity, personality that we've created for ourself. With this view comes a feeling of separation—reality is "in here" and future potentials all exist "out there."

But if we are to transform like the caterpillar into the butterfly, we have to realize that all possibilities lay within each of us.

In my case, I was like the regular cells in the caterpillar at first, just doing my job, just doing whatever was necessary to get through each day. I definitely had some "imaginal" in me, as I recognized the state of my pain was not sustainable and I attempted to define some vision of a new version of me. But it took some time before I could really organize my mind and all of my cells around that vision. When I reached my maximum capacity for pain and suffering, all of my pain cells began to die off and new cells began to form in an effort to promote this new, empowered, soaring-high-as-a-kite version of me. I had become the butterfly. And people noticed. My friends began to tell me that something shifted in me in a BIG way, in a very positive way. I became much lighter, I was pursuing my dreams, I believed in myself in a way they had never seen before; it was a complete metamorphosis.

I had absolutely no specifics about my future version of me when I first embarked on this journey, but I had very solid ideas, visions, and feelings about the general essence of what that would be, and that's where I started. I knew some of the characteristics and I could feel the corresponding emotions: I knew I wanted to help people. That had been a common theme my entire life. That would feel fulfilling. I knew I had some sort of message and wanted to speak it. I knew that the new version of me felt empowered. I knew I had gained a new kind of confidence, I no longer held any fear about failing. I knew that felt incredibly robust and assured. The beautiful thing was that the more I rested my attention on that future version, the more specifics came to me—in meditation, in dreams, during workouts, often seemingly randomly. Over time, I became the actor in the play, playing two roles and anticipating my own makeup change into another character, and it was truly fun! Now I envisioned myself writing books, speaking to crowds, helping others reach their goals, making incredible connections, and learning as much as I could. This never would have happened prior to July of 2014! Had I known about and believed in the possibilities, I would have begun this journey *years* ago!

For me, it took a serious injury for me to fully commit to my mind-set, my mental hygiene. I simply made the promise to heal my mind and not allow any negativity in. Never did I consider what it would lead to, nor did I contemplate how long it would take to cause my effect. I just promised myself that I would start, and take pleasure in, the practice. The rest unfolded from there.

I can't stress enough that you don't need to wait for an event, an injury, or an illness. The time is always now. And, just as importantly, you don't need anything external to happen. As health coaches, my colleagues and I often hear things like, "If my husband would just change his habits, I could do 'this,'" or, "If my wife doesn't support me, I can't do it." We don't need the approval or support of others, though, only our own approval and support.

Don't rush it. Just trust that it will come, because it is absolutely within you already, and most of all, have fun with it! Don't put any pressure on yourself, and if you feel like you are doing so, there is likely a limiting belief getting in your way, so congratulate yourself for identifying it! If you can't fully envision a new self, don't worry. Over time, you will re-connect with it, so just trust in that, because the answers are already and always have been within you.

Are you ready to undergo your makeup change, your mind redesign?

EXERCISE:

- Is there a dream you never chased, a better career, or some other opportunity you can envision? What are the characteristics? What are the associated emotions? Try jotting down the characteristics of the new job, the new you, the dream vacation, or whatever it is. Next, find a matching emotion to each.

Example: Dream Vacation

Characteristic	Emotion/Feeling
Cruise on open seas	Freedom, soothing
Socializing	Connected, fun
Around the world	Exciting, thrilling

CHAPTER TWENTY-TWO

BEING THE BUTTERFLY

"Know thyself, or at least keep
renewing the acquaintance."
-Robert Brault

After my brain injury, I had an amazing experience and reconnection—full, robust and true reconnection—with my true self once again, as if seeing an old friend and saying, "Oh, it's you!" I don't know for sure, but it is my belief that the forced state of meditation after the injury brought me to a greater state of consciousness and surrender that began this process. Since that event, I have let a lot of anger and anxiety go, fully releasing it al out of my mind and body. I no longer worry about anything. I no longer believe in lack. I no longer live in the memories of the past of my childhood. It is as if none of it even existed any longer, or ever did. Sure, I have memories, but no longer is there any energetic charge associated with them. Simply memories, neutral in emotional nature.

My world, my reality, was literally transformed when I became committed to my mental hygiene and began to improve my thoughts, attitudes, and beliefs. To many, my head injury was an awful, tragic event. To me, however, it just was what it was. It happened, and I could not change my new circumstances, but I most definitely had the power to change *my attitude about the circumstances,* and to learn and make something positive from it.

Throughout the healing process, I was tested: people who offered to help never showed, numerous doctors maintained my electrical nerve pain was in my head (but it was actually a consequence of the injury, and it took persistence on my part, and the eleventh or twelfth doctor finally took images that showed clearly what the problem was), I was overprescribed medication that left me suicidal, a particularly egocentric doctor told me that I needed to emotionally accept that I would have serious limitations for the rest of my life (I wasn't buying it), a second opinion urged that I needed another fusion and laminectomy STAT (wasn't buyin' that either), friends stopped talking to me during my worst days (a limiting belief they hold about pain, people in pain), and a number of other examples that would infuriate most. But these circumstances only made me dig in further. I was increasingly determined that no single circumstance, nor the collective, would define me as anything other than who I really am at my core. I was not about to become my injury.

I was 150% committed and the more I practiced, the better I felt, and the better I felt, the more I wanted to practice. And the more I practiced, the more I viewed my life as full and robust, and my days on earth like little presents I had the fortune of unwrapping each day. The happier I became, the more I paid attention. Now, at the time, I had no idea that there was actual *science* behind the tools I was developing and using. Later in the process, I learned the science behind why these tools worked so well for me. The magical thing was that I trusted that my mind and body knew what was best for me, and I paid attention. The ultimate result was a complete metamorphosis—I mean this was LIFE ALTERING!

Eventually, I drifted into a consistent state of bliss and happiness I've never experienced before, and I was, and still am, able to find joy even in the crummiest of situations. While I was in the process of writing this book, my father passed, my mother's health declined substantially, and my dog became terminally ill. I was notified that, as a result of a merger, my employment would probably not last more than a few months. Shortly following that, a physical injury happened. It was an extremely trying year and, had these events taken place five years prior, I'm sure I would have been devastated and depressed. But even through my father's passing, I found so much joy and appreciation. In my mother's post-stroke state of being, I found nothing but love and gratitude. Even with my job on the line, I had the inner knowing that all would be well. Of course, I still have my challenges—certain environments, for example, trigger my old mind, but I now have the tools to successfully address these challenges. Something happened during the healing process subsequent to my injury that altered me forever. I knew that, without a doubt, intuitively, but I had no idea about any science that might explain what exactly had altered me and my personality forever.

I still continue to experience numerous neurological, orthopedic and musculoskeletal symptoms and consequences of the injury. My vision and vestibular systems are still problematic. Because of the lack of harmony between those systems, frequent unpredictable and extreme dizziness can often make it challenging to sit, drive, or even drink a glass of water. The shifting and consequential fusion at L4/5 puts extra strain on the spine above and below. I continue to require routine therapies to address structural issues and some ongoing pain. Under elevated stress, I experience even additional symptoms. Meditation continues to be incredibly important in my recovery. I also continue to regularly practice the exercises I've included in this book, and to develop more.

Although I honor the need to feel grief or sadness when necessary, and just be human, I continue to smile in appreciation for every little gift I receive each and every day. The profound purpose and happiness I have found through my journey far outweighs any physical challenge. So, although I still have recovery to achieve, I am happy all the way through it. The injury never did, and does not now, define me. I was not then, and am not now, a victim. I am Lynn. Self-realized and self-actualizing Lynn. In a very strange yet magnificent way, my injury was a blessing.

Unfortunately, many of us wait until we are truly suffering to embark on a transformation. In my case, it was a serious, traumatic brain and spinal cord injury. But we do NOT have to wait for an illness, injury, or trauma to embark on this amazing journey. We are never too old, too young, too sick, too thin, too fat, too anything. We do not have to wait, and we don't even need a reason to improve our living by improving our thoughts. Why not be happier and more fulfilled, just because? You see, when you change your outlook on things, look out, because things are going to change!

I state often in the book that you need to do the work in order to experience this amazing transformation. A negative meaning is often assigned to the word "work," but I like to refer to it as W.O.R.K., Where Our Realities Kindle, because in doing the work is where our new reality begins to ignite. This is how I like to view perseverance, which includes practice without resistance. It is a knowing—when we know something to be true and we trust in it, then we continue to do the work, the practice without any resistance or opposition, just acceptance. It is not enough to do the exercises for six weeks, and then return to your familiar environment, your old habits and behaviors (triggered by your environment). It is not enough to practice for six weeks and then toss it to the side (although, the fact is, that if you do practice consistently for six weeks, you probably won't want to go back!). Your body and mind must be 100% on board and in alignment, and most importantly, you must believe in the possibilities. If you lack belief, trust me, that resistance will keep you from truly transforming. So believe in your future. You deserve the best experience this life has to offer you.

Will you have bad days? Sure. Of course, you will! But if you do the work, even the bad days won't be so bad. Doing the work is SO worth it, and YOU are worth it! Like the caterpillar who transforms from a ground species into a beautiful butterfly, flittering in the air, you will feel lighter, as if you have new wings. You will feel empowered, robust, confident, and in love with you! You will become the beautiful and divine creative being you came here to be and will want nothing more than to be YOU, because no one can do that as perfectly or as beautifully as you can.

You will no longer live conditionally, over-compromising yourself at the cost of yourself. You will no longer wait for something to materialize in order to feel bliss and happiness. You will no longer judge yourself or others. You will feel empowered. You will feel robust. You will be fearless! You will step into that divine creative genius that you are! You will ascend to a much higher state of mind and vibration. You will exude appreciation and positive energy, and people will take notice. You will feel true alignment and congruence of mind, heart, and body.

I'm so passionate about this work, and I'm so passionate about helping others experience their birthright of bliss. Too many of us are searching for answers, when the answers already reside within each of us already. It's just up to us to uncover and discover the power we hold.

ABOUT THE AUTHOR

LYNN DELGAUDIO

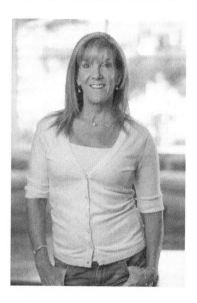

Lynn DelGaudio is an integrative health coach, motivational speaker, and author. After sustaining a traumatic brain injury in 2014, Lynn had to learn how to redesign her mind, literally. She now coaches individuals and companies on how to do the same. Whether you're an entrepreneur feeling stuck, a busy professional who wants a more creative, productive and fulfilling experience, or an employer who wishes the same for your team, Lynn has the tools to get you back on track, regain your balance and mojo, and create a more vibrant, inspired, productive, and empowered environment and life. She believes in the brilliant ability of the mind to catapult us into amazing places in our lives. You, too, can transform your life and redesign your mind with the techniques Lynn has to offer!

Made in the USA
Middletown, DE
19 May 2019